GOODBYE SKINNY

HELLO SIZE HEALTHY

A Woman's Guide To Becoming Healthy
Happy and Satisfied

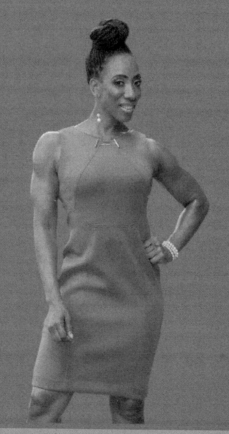

LATICIA " ACTION" JACKSON

Fitness Olympian, Women' s Health & Fitness Expert, MPH

Published in arrangement with
www.npoweredcoaching.com

By

Laticia "Action" Jackson
Fitness Olympian
5-Time N.P.C. Fitness Champion/IFBB Fitness Pro
Masters of Public Health (M.P.H.)
Certified Master Level Personal Trainer
Certified Lifestyle and Weight Management Specialists
Certified Corporate Wellness Coach
Voted "In Weekly's Best Trainer on The Gulf Coast 2016"

Layout, Edit, and Design © Goof Proof
www.goofproof.us

Fitness Images by Jiame Rivera
Jar Studio.com

Visit our website at
www.npoweredcoaching.com
or email us at npoweredcoaching@gmail.com

"Laticia "Action" Jackson is a student of the game and a master of her craft."

Daryl Haley ~ Retired N.F.L New England Patriots

"Laticia Jackson is a fitness inspiration who walks the walk.
Follow her lead and you're sure to change your body for the better."

Brad Schoenfeld, MS, CSCS ~ Author: Women's Home Workout Bible

"Undeniably the best fitness trainer I have ever had the privilege to interview
or work with. She pushes you to be your best. Not only physically- and believe
me she's tough. But internally which gives you the permission to be your best-
mind, body and spirit!"

Mark Mathis ~ CW31 Good Day Sacramento

"One Dynamic Lady... whose passion to succeed and make a difference has
made her dynamic in all areas of her life."

Mike Lackner ~ Body Fitness-UK

"Every workout was earnest, extremely enjoyable and tailored to my personal
needs allowing me to reach my maximum physical fitness level. Laticia was
inspirational, motivating and I highly endorse her as a physical fitness trainer
for anyone and everyone."

Lloyd C. ~ Colonel U.S.A.F., Dayton Ohio

"Working with Laticia Jackson as my personal trainer has been an empowering
experience. She trains your body to achieve maximum performance, teaches
your mind new fitness concepts and encourages your inner self to embrace
and love the healthy person you are destined to be."

Sandra H. ~ California Police Dept., Sacramento, CA

Contents

~ ~ ~

On this fitness journey,
I challenge you
to define the true
meaning of beauty,
get into the best shape
of your life and
to live your life
with purpose.

~ ~ ~

This book is dedicated to every woman who desires the world to recognize her external beauty, but to also acknowledge her character, intelligence and moral values. This book is also dedicated to the women who have shared their stories of self-discovery with me. You know who you are.

I am forever grateful to you for your truth and transparency. Your honesty and willingness to share your experiences with me has given me the courage to share my insecurities with the world and not be ashamed. My internal struggles have taught me many valuable lessons, and one of the most valuable lessons I have learned is that in order for one to be fit on the outside, one must first be fit from an internal perspective. Unfortunately, this isn't a concept taught often to women in today's society.

Instead of women being taught to value themselves for internal and moral reasons, they are constantly led to believe their value is measured by their appearance - including the shape of their body. Trying to measure up to these unrealistic expectations has the ability to create feelings of inadequacies, low self-worth and low self-esteem in women and young girls.

Therefore, in the following pages, it is my intention to encourage women to reject the current social norm and to search for a deeper meaning of what it means to be beautiful and fit.

This fitness training book doesn't emphasize skinny - it emphasizes healthy from a mental, physical and emotional standpoint. What good is a flat stomach if you don't love yourself?

On the following pages, you will find amazing tools to get you into the best shape of your life, and you will learn how to live your life with purpose while being fit, healthy and happy.

It is my hope that the words on the following pages will give women of all races and backgrounds the inspiration to love themselves, the courage to unlock their inner strength and the knowledge to become a healthier, happier, more fit version of who they were created to become.

You're a precious jewel, and it's time for you to shine. Are you ready?

Stay Fit,

Stay True,

Stay You!

Laticia

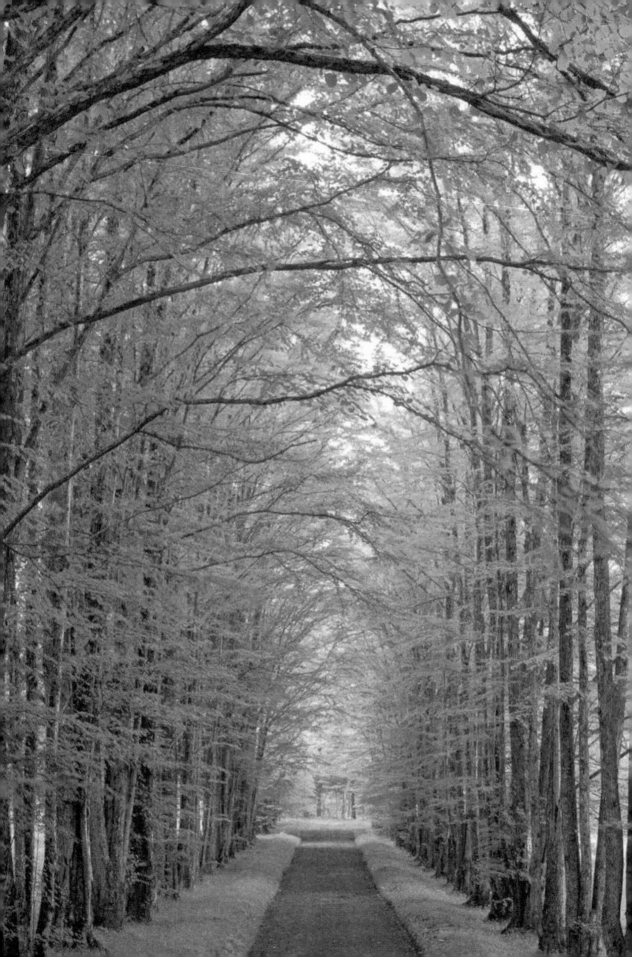

Learning to love myself has been a continual process with many painful destinations. I have learned many valuable lessons on this journey and one of the most valuable lessons I have learned is that in order for one to become fit on the outside, one must first nourish their internal well-being. My journey of self-love and self-discovery has caused me to look deep within myself in order to challenge the pain of abandonment, feelings of rejection and address the continual need to prove my self-worth through my accomplishments.

Making the decision to peel away my layers of hurt has given me the freedom to share my pain and discoveries with the world and not feel ashamed. Therefore, it is my hope that by being vulnerable with you, in return you will look within yourself and begin your journey to learning to love yourself and realize that being fit goes beyond the size of your clothing, the number on a scale and toned arms.

How did my journey begin?

I grew up in a very loving and nourishing home with a strong bond between my two older sisters and my parents. Without warning, this bond was destroyed when my parents divorced after 20 years of marriage. At the vulnerable age of 12, I didn't know why their marriage ended, but I knew the place I once called home would never be the same. My dad left and I never knew why, the only thing I knew was that I no longer felt safe. Once he left, he was no longer a regular part of my life and his absence hurt me tremendously. His absence left a hole in my heart and I began to believe if I were good enough he would have stayed with me and my family.

Although growing up my mother showered me with love, and reaffirmed I wasn't the cause of my father's leaving, the emptiness from my dad leaving lingered in my heart for many years to come.

As I grew older, I carried anger in my heart towards my dad for leaving me. The anger in my heart caused me to struggle with trusting others, especially men. As a result of this pain, I built an emotional wall around my heart keeping everyone at bay. I was determined to never allow another man to hurt or abandon me, therefore, I made a vow to myself that I would be successful and not depend on anyone, especially a man. In my mind my emotional wall would protect me, but it didn't. I was on an emotional ride that I wouldn't get off until years to come.

In 1999, I entered the United States Air Force, where I graduated with honors from Basic Military Training (B.M.T.). I was one out of five people in a squadron of 200 to earn this title. From there I went on to attend Air Force Technical Training School, where I graduated in the top ten percent of my class and was eventually stationed at Randolph Air Force Base, TX, which was a Head Quarters Unit as a result of my honor status. It was during this time that I began weight training and fell passionately in love with the body and fitness after an encounter with a local celebrity bodybuilder. This local bodybuilder noticed my genetic potential and offered to train me for my first fitness competition.

After six months of intense fitness training, I entered and won my very first fitness competition. Needless to say, I was hooked on fitness and couldn't turn back. My placement for a beginner in my sport was an amazing accomplishment that grabbed the attention of many fitness magazines and nutrition sponsors. The night of my win I celebrated, but the excitement of my win and new-found passion was shortly lived. I was proud of myself but didn't feel complete. Although I took home the highest placement, my father wasn't there and I needed to hear that he was proud me. These words never came and wouldn't come until years later, and so the perfectionist cycle of trying to prove my worth through my accomplishments continued.

> ## I was hurting inside and searching for belonging.

While in the military, I began dating and my dating life became just like everything else in my life - chaotic. My relationships became just as unhealthy as my need for approval. While in the military, I found myself in a relationship with a man eleven years older than I was. Due to my fear of abandonment, I had to be with him at all times and constantly needed to know he cared. I was co-dependent and over time, this relationship became unhealthy and I left. Years later I would find myself in similar unhealthy relationships, mainly with older men. At the time, I thought it was just the type of men I was meeting and had nothing to do with me. Unfortunately, I wasn't aware of my own behavior and unhealthy choices in men. Unknowingly, I was seeking the love my father never gave me from my relationships.

I was hurting inside and searching for belonging and clung to the person I was

in a relationship with even if it didn't feel right. I needed and wanted to be loved. I wanted to be loved so badly that having a little love seemed better than not being loved at all. Although this behavior was obvious to others and not to myself, I am grateful my creator had better plans for me.

One day a friend invited me to church where I heard the message of God's love. I wanted to be loved so desperately that I was drawn to this message. On this day, I allowed God into my heart but the pain of abandonment and rejection continued.

I continued competing as an amateur fitness competitor for a couple of years, and in 2006 I went on to earn my title as an International Federation of Body Building and Fitness Professional (I.F.B.B.). Being one of the world's top professional fitness competitors opened doors for me to be featured in nationally-publicized fitness magazines such as Oxygen, Muscle and Fitness Hers, Flex and many more. One would be ecstatic for these opportunities, but this wasn't my experience. When I was featured in any fitness publication, the only thing I could focus on was the imperfect pictures of myself. Instead of celebrating a successful moment, I needed to look perfect and would be disappointed for days and not share the magazines with friends and families if I didn't believe I looked perfect.

This cycle of being a perfectionist transferred to other areas of my life, including my academics. In 2004, I graduated with a degree in Human Performance with a 3.5 G.P.A.. Every semester during this time I made the Dean's List, but I would always miss the President's List by a point or two. This did not sit well with me and I was determined with my next degree to do better. During this time, I was inducted into Phi Theta Kappa Honor Society but I still wasn't satisfied, regardless of how well I did. In my mind's eye I had to do better and eventually I would realize how valuable I was to my dad and everyone else.

Therefore, in 2006 I went on to earn my second degree in Exercise Science from the University of West Florida where I graduated with a 3.6 GPA and made it into the International Honor Society. Once again these accolades were great, but weren't good enough to make me feel complete. I felt the need to do more to prove my worth and just maybe I would hear those long awaited words from my father. I was on a vicious cycle with no signs of stopping.

In 2006, while finishing my second degree, I met a man who would eventually become my husband. He was articulate, handsome, charming, and attentive. After nine months of dating; I became his wife. During our courtship, there were signs of jealousy and controlling behavior, but I had finally found someone who in my mind loved me and I couldn't let him go. I believed I was going to finally get the love my father never gave me, but this was one of the biggest mistakes of my life.

After we were married, he would often tell me I was his property and that I belonged to him. I couldn't be alone without him and at all times he had to know my whereabouts. Due to his controlling behavior, I began to lose my smile, my laughter and my joy, the true essence of who I am. There were nights after having fights and being called vulgar names, I would cry out to God to help me get out of this situation. I was being both verbally and physically abused, but no one knew about it. My thought process at the time was very unhealthy. I would say to myself, "How can a woman who is educated, fit, and successful who has it all together be going through this?" I felt no one could know about my abuse, I was afraid if people knew, they would think I was unsuccessful and weak-minded for allowing such behaviors to occur.

Finally on September 17, 2007, the silence of my abuse was broken. After a jealous rage, my ex-husband grabbed me by my neck and proceeded to choke me. As I looked into his angered eyes, seconds seemed like hours as my breath became more and more shallow. Just before I passed out, he released his hands from around my neck, slapped my face and called me a vulgar name. He walked away in a casual manner as if nothing had transpired.

He fled the scene and a day later the police found him and charged him with attempted murder. These charges were eventually dropped to domestic violence charges due to my choosing to not attend his court hearing. The day he was arrested, I was in such an unhealthy state of mind, I called the police wanting to know if he was OK. You may ask, "Didn't this person attempt to take your life?" To do such a thing only affirmed that I was emotionally ill. The cop whom I spoke with during this call was baffled that I called to check on my ex-husband. His tone and response reflected disbelief that I would call. Days after this incident occurred, I was finally in a safe environment. Once I settled in, I knew it was time to get honest with myself and I had to address the root cause of my issues.

> Regardless of a woman's appearance and the size of her body, the true essence of who she is lives within.

Although acknowledging my behavior was a harsh reality, it was time to deal with my underlining hurt and pain. If not, I would eventually continue my negative patterns of behavior that would lead to self-destruction and possibly death.

....

We live in a society where women are chasing fictionalized images of beauty and unrealistic notions of perfection.

....

In the blink of an eye, I realized my life could have been lost. From that moment on, I knew I had to get real with myself and address my internal issues. Regardless of how fit my body was, I was unfit on the inside. Going through domestic abuse was a life-changing experience, but I was determined not to become a victim in this situation. Therefore, I had to accept the decision I made to marry someone who I knew was jealous and controlling. I couldn't blame him for everything - I had to take ownership of my part as well. I was fully aware that the pain from my father leaving me at an early age affected me, but I didn't want to blame my father for all of my actions and decisions.

The first step in my healing process was to admit that I was in pain and needed help. Through God's love and family support, I began to heal and eventually was able to forgive my ex-husband. I realized that hurt people often hurt others and in many ways he too was hurting. It was also painful to accept that for years I was hiding my pain behind my accomplishments. I wanted to get better; so I continued to uncover the truth of who I had become. Since that time, I have worked hard to address the issue of being a perfectionist, overachiever and many other internal issues. I realize that I will always be driven, but my self-worth is no longer dictated by my accomplishments.

I no longer need to be in a relationship with a man to feel secure about myself. I desire a healthy relationship, but don't need to be in one to feel great about who I am. Now, I take time every day to work on the internal side of who I am and treasure the woman I have become. I have forgiven my father for leaving me and our relationship is work in progress. He is now a more regular part of my life and it feels great to have him around. Having my dad in my life has allowed some of my old wounds to heal from years of pain and rejection, but to say I am 100 percent recovered from years of emotional baggage from his leaving isn't the truth. I am still a work in progress and open to seeking the truth behind my pain.

I am currently earning a Master's Degree in Public Health, but this time around I am not earning my degree to prove my self-worth. I am earning my degree in order to educate and empower people to change their lives by taking control of their health.

Why did I share my story?

I shared my story due to the fact that today we live in a society where women are chasing fictionalized images of beauty and unrealistic notions of perfection. We are often led to believe if we look perfect, act perfect and have size zero bodies, then our lives will be perfect. I am here to dispel this falsity.

I am educated, fit and wear a size 4 clothing, been featured in fitness magazines around the world and in many ways successful, yet I wasn't exempt from pain, insecurities or disappointment.

Like many of you, I have covered my pain with success, accomplishments and my appearance. Maybe you cover your pain by overeating, or binging and purging, or maybe you cover your pain by purchasing the most expensive clothes to create an image for the world. It doesn't matter how you cover your pain, we all have it and if we are honest with ourselves, at some point in life, we have worn masks to hide the pain.

I am forever grateful for my pain based on the reality that pain has taught me things that joy never could. I am the woman I am today because of my pain and if my story can inspire someone and help them avoid some of my pitfalls, then my pain wasn't in vain.

The woman I see today continues to make self-improvements daily, but overall is happy, healthy and empowered.

I have shared my story in order to prove to the world that regardless of a woman's appearance and the size of her body, the true essence of who she is lives within.

~ ~ ~

I am forever thankful for my pain based on the reality that pain has taught me things joy never could.

~ ~ ~

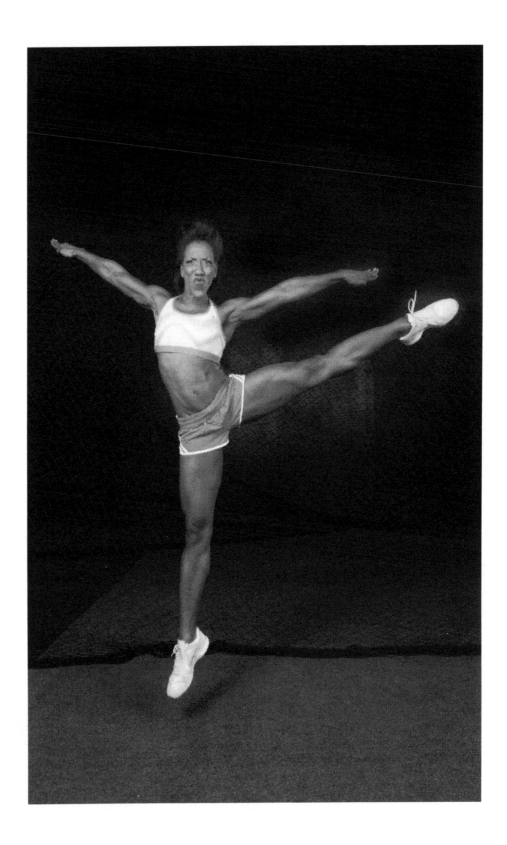

Acknowledgments

First and most importantly, I would like to thank my Creator, Jesus Christ for entrusting me with this vision. I am forever grateful for the gifts you have given me. May I always live a life that is pleasing and honorable in your sight. Without you, I would not have had the strength to endure this process. I love you and will always need you. You are sources of where I gain all of my power.

Mom, there are not enough words in the dictionary to describe how much I love you. Regardless of what life has brought my way, you have always been there to love me through my trials. A day without you is comparable to a day without the sun. I pray that one day I will be a great mother just like you. I miss our girl nights out and spending quality time with you.

Dad, you have always been a silent strength in my life. I have inherited your tremendous work ethic and it has paid off in so many ways. You are a man of great character and integrity and I pray to one day marry a man with your morals and values. I look forward to our relationship growing. It's great to find out who I get my long arms from!

Yolanda, I would like to thank you for always being there for me. You are always just a call away. You are officially my human resource person. Your strength as a soldier, mother, sister, wife and friend is encouraging. May God give you all the desires of your heart and much more. I pray you learn to laugh more often; you know I do enough laughing for the both of us. You are a great big sister and I love you.

Shanta, we have been friends for as long as I can remember. Even though you have left me outside in the cold to get a donut, I will always love you. You are the true image of a wife and mother. You are selfless and I admire that about you. Your constant prayers, love and encouragement is priceless. You have a special place in my heart. I love you butterfly. Thanks for letting me be your little sister.

Dr. Niza Berry. My bestie for life! You are perfect for me. You have helped me realize how valuable I am. You have stuck by me in some of the hardest and darkest times in life and for that I am thankful. We will have lots of stories to tell me children and your nieces and nephews! Thank you for loving me just the way I am!

To my nieces and nephews, you bring so much joy to my life. It has been such a pleasure to be your auntie. Seeing each of you grow up brings joy to my heart. I love each of you.

To my brother-in-laws, thanks for loving my sisters and being great men.

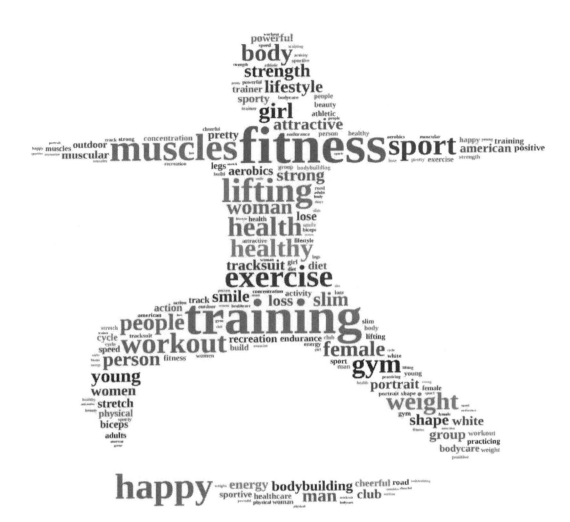

Let your fitness journey begin!

In today's society, women are constantly bombarded with unattainable images of beauty and bodily perfection. These images are seen on infomercials, billboards and in magazines that flaunt women who are either a size zero or size small, leaving women comparing their bodies to the women they see in these advertisements. The bombardments of these images often leave women feeling self-conscience about their own bodies and appearance. Unattainable and fictionalized images of bodily perfection have also created insecurities in young girls as young as five who believe they are fat. Why should a five year old be consumed with her weight? The media and society has created a size game and as women it's time to stop playing this game.

The size game is over and it's time for women to learn how to embrace their bodies, learn the tools to become healthier and discover how to love themselves whether they are a size 6 or 16 and *I'm Not a Size Zero-Defining Your Curves While Loving Yourself* is the tool to help women accomplish this.

I'm Not a Size Zero, Defining Your Curves While Loving Yourself is a fitness-training workbook that emphasizes being fit isn't about being a size small, it's about being a size healthy. Unlike many fitness training books that emphasize just the physical aspect of a woman, *I'm Not a Size Zero* emphasizes that creating a strong, functional, toned body first starts with self–acceptance and being emotionally fit from an inner perspective. Teaching women how to accept and love themselves has the ability to increase confidence and the sense of empowerment to change their bodies and their lives.

In the following chapters, you will be encouraged to define your true meaning of beauty, what it means to be fit and discover why in the past you haven't accomplished your fitness goals.

Therefore, before you begin with the first chapter, ask yourself:

Why are you taking this fitness journey?

Your success on this journey will be heavily dependent on how you answer this question.

As you take this journey, it is important to make this journey about yourself and no one else. As women, we often make changes for other people, peer and societal pressures and not for ourselves. Without the belief and conviction that you are worth getting fit, you may find yourself struggling to reach your fitness destination, especially if you are taking this journey for someone else.

On this fitness adventure, you will learn how to recognize the emotional barriers that may have prevented you from previous success, how to set fitness goals, train for your body type, easy to learn resistance and cardiovascular training techniques and fit girl's gym etiquette.

Learning sound nutritional principals is essential to creating the fit body you desire, therefore you will be provided with a comprehensive explanation of macro-nutrients (protein, fat, carbohydrates) and learn how to incorporate these nutrients into your daily meal plan. You will be provided with quick and easy palate pleasing recipes for breakfast, lunch and dinner that will entice your palate and encourage you to become creative in the kitchen.

Remember, getting fit is a lifetime commitment and you are worth the time and effort it will take to reach your destination. If you are ready to stop playing the size game and get healthy, then string up your Nike's and let's do it!

~ ~ ~

The size game is over
and it's time
for women to learn
how to embrace
their bodies,
learn the tools
to become healthier,
and discover how
to love themselves
whether they
are a size 6 or 16.

~ ~ ~

Part I

Are You Ready to Love Yourself Fit?

Love Yourself Fit

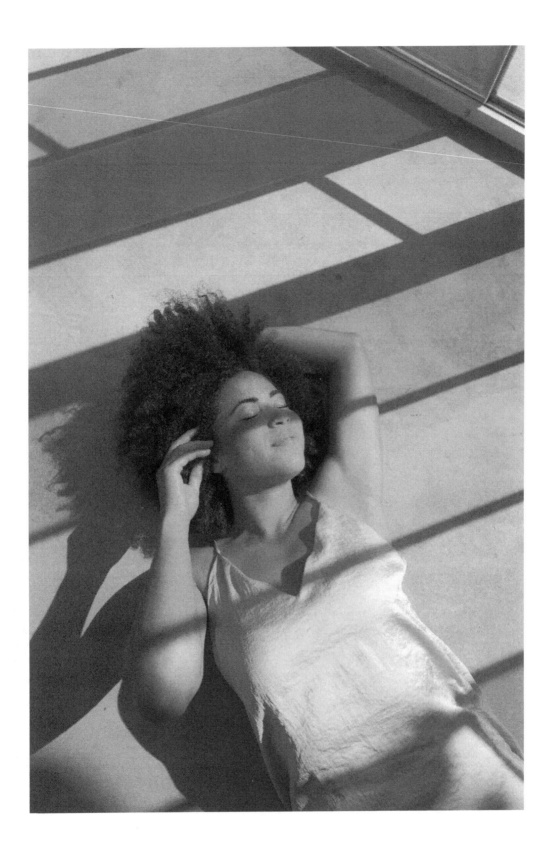

Chapter

The media doesn't know you, so why give them so much power over you?

1

The Subliminal Message

The Subliminal Message

Today we live in a society where women are constantly bombarded by commercials, magazines and advertisements that flaunt images of unrealistic bodily perfection. These images attempt to convince women that if they have shinier hair, wrinkle-free skin and toned size zero bodies, then their lives will be perfect. Have you bought into this message? If so, why?

> When was the last time you saw a commercial advertising products that enhance your inner beauty?

Why is there such a driving force behind our journey to unreachable perfection? Why are we seeking a constantly-changing illusion and then chase this illusion, failing to realize it is unrealistic and unattainable?

Has chasing the illusion of bodily perfection helped contribute to eating disorders (bulimia and anorexia nervosa) of approximately seven million women and left our young girls as young as 5 dieting? Yes, I said dieting. Young girls who see images of thinness and who have mothers who experience negative feelings regarding their own bodies begin to emulate negative body issues themselves. In many ways, this behavior can lead to other negative eating and exercise patterns as these young girls become adolescents and young adults. If you're a mother, it is essential to understand that your daughters will learn either positive or negative body images based on what they learn from you. Therefore, it is time for you to start loving yourself and your body. Don't allow the size of your clothing or the number on the scale dictate your worth.

Although you may feel alone and believe you are the only woman who feels unhappy with her body, you aren't alone. Women of all ages experience the effects of the media's portrayal of bodily perfection and beauty. No woman is exempted from these pressures.

Just count the number of commercials and advertisements that are directed at women. How can we not feel these pressures? We can't hide from society, but we can make the decision to not allow the media to dictate our worth by the size of our bodies. I am not expressing that being unhealthy is acceptable, what I am expressing is we as women have to make the decision that our worth isn't determined by what society calls beautiful.

Aren't you tired of chasing the unattainable illusion of bodily perfection and desire to get for all the right reasons? If you are, don't waste another day consumed by images of digitally perfected bodies. Start embracing your body today and become fit for all the right reasons.

Become Fit For All the Right Reasons

Become fit for more than vanity reasons: If you are only losing weight to fit into a swimsuit or go to a special event, your weight loss will not be permanent. Choose your health over vanity and it will last longer.

Do not compare yourself to others: You are fearfully and wonderfully made. Comparing your body to other women will leave you feeling insecure about yourself. Embrace yourself and become a fitter version of who you were created to be.

Do not believe the hype: The images of women in health and fitness magazines do not represent the average size woman. Being a size healthy is more important than any other size.

Believe you are worth it: Regardless of your size, believe you are worth the time, effort and money required to become fit. Make fit look good on you!

Identify your internal greatness: Often times women focus solely on improving their outer appearance and neglect their inner spirit. Discover at least five great inner qualities that make you a great woman.

Compliment yourself: Every day is a chance to re-affirm how great you are. Do not wait to drop a size before you compliment yourself.

A Billion Dollar Industry

Have you ever flipped through a women's health or fitness magazine and envied the body of a beautiful model? Besides her toned body, an ad guarantees a body like hers if you simply use the product she uses. After looking at her picture, you may have wanted to go and hide in your baggiest pair of sweats and eat your favorite ice cream. Have you ever felt this way? If you have, it's easy to understand why.

The fitness and diet related industry does not connect with the average size woman who is a size 12-14. The pages of many women's health and fitness magazines are saturated with unhealthy diet products and images of thin women subliminally putting pressure on all women who read these magazines to be thin.

Recently while reading a women's fitness magazine, I came across an ad that grabbed my attention. It was an ad for protein and it read, "When you hit the gym you workout hard for ONE reason, to look sexy outside the gym." I asked myself; _"Have I trained over ten years just to look sexy outside the gym?"_ No, being sexy is not the _only_ reason I exercise or train.

I'm not saying that being in shape won't make you feel sexy, but being sexy isn't the only reason women workout. Women workout for a myriad of reasons - such as having functional strength to accomplish everyday tasks like carrying groceries or lifting their children out of their car seats. Women exercise to create strong bones that ward off osteoporosis and other muscular debilitating ailments. We exercise to feel strong, empowered and accomplished.

**"Shut out the narrative of being thin!"**

Why is thin such a craze and how will the average size woman measure up to these images?

They won't and neither should they try.

Every woman's body structure is unique and it's time for women to stop comparing their body to unrealistic images. Regardless of how much the diet and fitness industry pushes women to fit into a mold, every woman wasn't created to be thin and curves are a beautiful asset. If you are going to get fit, you have to stop comparing your body to other women, especially women in magazines. You are smart and realize there isn't a diet pill to substitute for hard work and discipline in and out the gym.

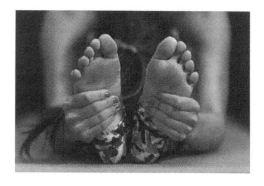

You can spend thousands of dollars trying to force your body to do something it was never created to do or you can accept your body and learn how to eat healthy and exercise properly for your specific body type. Aren't you ready to embrace your body and define what fit means to you on your own terms?

It is vital for you to know that whether you are a size 6 or 16, taking responsibility for your health should make you feel sexy. Working hard to create the body you desire will bring confidence and a sense of fulfillment that no one can give you. You will never find this confidence in a bottle of diet pills or anywhere else. Therefore, the next time you pick up a women's fitness or health magazine, do not compare yourself to another woman, you are a masterpiece and it's time for you to start believing it.

The Media's Effect on Women and Young Girls

Numerous studies show young girls and women are dissatisfied with their bodies and take drastic measures to become thin. Unrealistic body images shown in the media has helped contribute to many women having low self-esteem and negative body image issues. Some women manifest their dissatisfaction of their body by either starving themselves, becoming excessive exercisers and compulsive dieters. These unhealthy behaviors can lead to permanent health problems and in some cases, death. Therefore it is important to seek medical attention if you or someone you know is suffering with an eating disorder or other unhealthy behaviors. Don't be afraid to reach out for help - you are not alone.

Learn the signs of anorexia and bulimia.

Signs and Symptoms of Anorexia

- Persistent Denial

- Excessive amount of weight loss in a short period of time

- Preoccupation with calorie counting

- Excessive exercise patterns

- Changes in mood

- Distorted body image (falsely believing you are fat)

- Intense and exaggerated fears of gaining weight or becoming fat

- Refusal of food even when hungry

- Decrease in self-esteem and self-confidence

- Strong feeling of being in control of oneself

- Frequent arguments with others regarding food

- Increase in body hair (body hair acts as an heat insulator)

- Irregular menstrual cycles

Bulimia and anorexia nervosa are both life-threatening disorders. If you or someone you know have any signs or symptoms of bulimia or anorexia, please seek medical attention

Health Problems Associated with Anorexia

- Changes in metabolism

- Drop in blood pressure

- Fluctuating body temperatures, dizziness and weakness from malnutrition

- Heart complications

- Excessive storage of body fat

- The body "feeding" on itself

- Vitamin and mineral deficiency

- Death

Signs and Symptoms of Bulimia

- Patterns of secretly eating large amounts of food followed by purging

- Abuse of laxatives, diuretics or excessive exercise

- Feelings of isolation

- Decreased enjoyment of friendships

- Increase in mood swings

- Intense fears of becoming fat

- Feeling of loneliness and helplessness

- Decrease in self-esteem and self confidence

- Distorted body image (falsely believing you are fat)

Health Problems Associated with Bulimia

- Hair loss

- Dental problems

- Erosion of the esophagus

- Stomach and digestive problems

- Heart complications

- Dehydration

- Electrolyte imbalances, low potassium

- Death

The following website offers information and support groups for individuals with anorexia and bulimia.

www.nationaleatingdisorders.org

The Quest for the Perfect Body

The numbers below represent the amount of surgical procedures women elect to have on an annual basis. Could societal pressures lead women to augment their bodies in order to achieve the look of a *Perfect* Body?

What does the perfect body really look like?

Top Five Cosmetic Surgical Procedures (Annually):

Breast Augmentation (307,000)

Liposuction (218,000)

Nose Reshaping (204,000)

Eyelid Surgery (190,000)

Tummy Tuck (117,000)

(Source: American Society of Plastic Surgery)

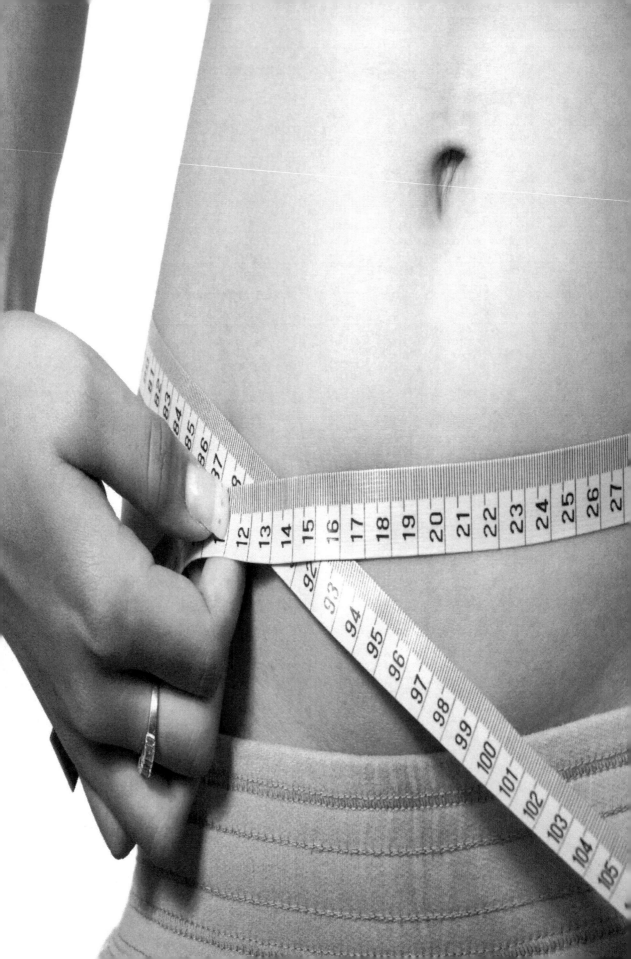

Chapter

You can't change yesterday, but you can change today!

2

A New Day, A New You

Take Off the Mask

It is no secret that everyone wants to be accepted, and as women we are taught the more physically attractive we are the more appealing we are to the world and to the opposite sex. As women, one way we attempt to receive acceptance is by creating a fictitious persona and the perfect body. Our fictitious persona and perfect bodies sometimes are created to cover up failures, insecurities, past hurts or shattered dreams. Ask yourself if this describes you.

If so, how long will you stay behind your mask?

In order to become healthy from an internal and external perspective, you will be required to look deep within yourself and uncover some truths. For many years I hid my insecurities behind my accomplishments and education. Maybe you have gained weight to cover up your fear of being rejected. Or maybe you keep your appearance perfect at all times to cover up your insecurities of not being accepted if you're flawed. Getting fit first starts with looking deeper than the external person you have created with superficial truths. Once you unveil your true self, people will see your authenticity - in return this will give you the freedom to accept yourself for who you really are apart from the image you may have created. What good is a flat stomach and toned arms when you really don't know who you are? Therefore, it's time to step away from your masks; you are no longer

auditioning for a play. Will the real you stand up?

The Audition is Over

Removing the masks you've worn for so long can be difficult, yet stepping away from your mask is necessary in order to reveal a true reflection of yourself. Deciding to let go of old behaviors can result in many personal challenges that may have prevented you from reaching your fitness goals in the past. Addressing these challenges may not be easy, but in the long run will be worth it. Maybe you have believed your marital relationship ended because you put on too much weight and your husband was no longer attracted to you. Or just maybe you believe you would get more acceptance from those around you if you lost more weight. Whatever internal issues you have dealt with in the past have to be brought into the light for your healing to begin.

Sometimes our bodies are the greatest testament of how we feel about ourselves on the inside. We often neglect this aspect of who we are. It is essential to understand that your body won't change until your mind changes how you see yourself.

Remove the Disguise

Share your fears and failures with a trustworthy source: When we feel safe, we are more willing to open up and share our true feelings. If you suffer from low self-esteem, eating problems or other issues, find someone you can confide in and admit to these issues.

Do not be afraid to admit you do not have it all together: Admitting that you don't have it all together takes pressure off of having to always be on top of everything. Release yourself from a perfectionist's mentality and ask for help when needed. Stop wearing the perfectionist mask.

Admit your weaknesses--we all have them: Once we acknowledge our weak areas, we can acquire tools to help improve in these areas. Acknowledging your weaknesses is a sign of growth and a desire for change.

Ask for help when you need it; you cannot conquer the world alone: Inviting someone to help you with your daily load can open more time for self-reflection and self-improvement, including working out more often. Asking for help is a sign of strength, not weakness.

Do not hide from your past, acknowledge your mistakes and move forward: Experience can be a great teacher if you allow it to teach you. The mistakes of your past are gone; do not allow them to hinder you from moving into your future.

Do not be afraid to be yourself. You are amazing: You're an amazing woman and have amazing qualities. Accept your greatness and continue to become a better version of yourself and don't base your worth on the size of your body.

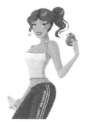

FIT JEWEL

True freedom is allowing yourself to become the best you!

Stranger in the Midst

You are slowly removing your mask and you're not content with what you are discovering. Years have gone by and you may have gotten married, changed jobs, given birth or completed your education and you discover you're not happy with yourself. Although you are grateful for your life experiences, your day-to-day routine has become taxing and you have forgotten about yourself. You're exhausted and in many ways feel like you're losing yourself. Your body has changed and you don't like what you're seeing.

One day while waiting in the grocery store checkout line, you notice a women's fitness magazine and on the cover is a youthful woman with abs of steal and an amazing backside. You begin to reflect. You remember the days when you were in better shape and felt great about yourself. What happened to those days? Why do those days seem so far in the distance? How did you let yourself go? Why didn't someone tell you that you weren't the same?

Slow down, exhale, it's never too late to change.

Superwoman Isn't Your Name

If you have ever felt the need to shout, "I need time for myself," welcome to the Superwoman Club. As women, we often find ourselves taking care of others as if it is programmed into our DNA and saying "no" is a cardinal sin. When we don't say no, we often find ourselves overwhelmed, overworked and overweight. On the other end of the spectrum, when we finally decide to make time for ourselves, the feelings of guilt and selfishness takes over. Let me tell you a little secret, come a little closer. It's perfectly acceptable to take off your Superwoman cape for an hour or two a day in order to do something healthy for yourself. If you don't take care of yourself, how can you take care of anyone else?

Do you take time for yourself?

Do you tell yourself someday you will get back to you?

That someday is now.

Have you been telling yourself that one day you are going to get back to exercising and eating healthier? If this is you, that someday is today!

Making a renewed commitment to yourself doesn't mean you have to look like the fitness models in the magazines, but it is possible to create a new and improved version of yourself. Do you want to have more energy to play with your children? Or what about fitting back into that dress you wore on your first date with your husband?

So how do you get back on track to making necessary changes? I am glad you asked.

Get Back on Track

The first step is to acknowledge what you do not like about yourself. This may sound contradictory to the purpose of this book, but it's not to belittle you - rather it's a part of the self-reflection process. Once this task is completed, ask yourself on a scale of 0-10 (0 low- 10 high) how willing, able and confident you are to address these issues. From there, determine the steps needed to make your desired changes. Be patient and kind with yourself and realize it will take time to make a change. Focus on the process versus the outcome, approaching your change in this manner will make the process more enjoyable and less overwhelming.

Secondly, establish a support system and communicate your needs and challenges. Sometimes making a change requires guidance and support. Requesting help and support is not a sign of weakness but a sign of strength. When you acknowledge the need for help, you begin to realize you can delegate your responsibilities and give up the need to be Superwoman. If you have gained weight and need further assistance to get you on the right track, review your budget to see if you can afford a personal trainer or gym membership. If this isn't feasible, there are several options such as community recreation centers or churches that offer free fitness programs. If you can't fit a trainer into your budget, you can purchase or rent workout videos for home, workout at the park or go for regular walks around your neighborhood. Encourage your husband/significant other to help around the house so you have more time for yourself. If time permits, create a fitness regimen for both of you. This will offer one-on-one time to build team work and spend valuable time together.

Last and most importantly, believe you have the ability to change whatever it is that you don't like. Believing in yourself will give you the motivation to keep going when times become rough and not beat yourself up in the process. Although change is challenging, we can't change what we are not willing to address.

Make Time for Yourself

- Find a special quiet place in your home that is off limits during your quiet time. Make it comfortable with a nice chair and pillows. Take this time to reflect and relax.

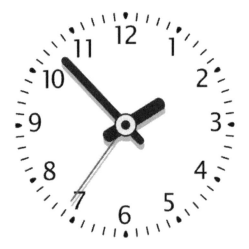

- Take 15-20 minutes a day to meditate or pray.
- Once a week take a hot bubble bath. Do not forget your aromatherapy candles and soft music.
- Schedule and write in your planner at least three days per week to exercise. Unless there is an

emergency do not miss your appointment.

- Do not be afraid to say no. You are one person and cannot take care of the entire world. The world will continue to function without you being involved in every aspect of life.
- Once a month, have a personal night out. It is always great to have a night where you can unwind and relax with your friends.
- Laugh aloud. Laughter is medicine for the soul.
- Don't take yourself so seriously. If you make a mistake or things do not turn out the way you want them to, evaluate the situation take necessary steps to prevent them from occurring again and move on.
- Every day, tell yourself how wonderful you are. If you can't speak positive affirmations to yourself, why should anyone else?

No More Excuses

Do you continually set fitness goals and don't follow through? Have you allowed things in your life to take priority over your health and you keep telling yourself tomorrow I'll start again but when tomorrow gets here, you have other excuses?

If you have allowed this to happen don't beat yourself up - but it's time to make your health a priority and let go of any and all excuses. Therefore, in order to move forward with your fitness goals it is important to identify the potential excuses that are holding you back. Do you lack team support from a friend or spouse? Do you lack the financial resources to start eating healthier? Whatever your excuses/challenge(s) are, discover a way(s) to resolve them.

I often like to say committing to your health is very similar to a relationship. There are good days and bad days, but you are in it for the long haul, you don't allow excuses to get in your way to having a meaningful relationship. The same goes for your health. If you are committed to getting healthier, put all your efforts into reaching and maintaining your fitness/health goals. No more excuses. Today is a new day and it's time to stop looking back and move forward.

Is there something that is holding you back from accomplishing your goals?

Have you attempted to get fit in the past and failed? If, so has this made you doubtful that you can follow through?

Do you lack a support system?

Age is Not an Excuse

For many women, age has become a logical reason as to why they aren't getting into shape and from different sources this belief is validated. The media is popular for subliminally telling women that when they reach a certain age, it's all downhill from there. This is far from the truth.

Have you reached an age in life where you think it's all downhill from where you are and you have given up trying to have a fit body at your age?

If you feel this way, you need to know age literally is just a number. There's no denying that as women age it's harder for them to get into shape, but it's not impossible.

Do not allow this mentality to prevent you from reaching your fitness goals.

If you feel it is too late, meet Sandra.

At the age of forty-eight, Sandra weighed over 200 pounds, was isolated and not living a very adventurous life. After a regular visit to her doctor, she realized she was tired of literally being tired and it was time to do something about her health.

She began making small steps, such as making wiser food choices, then eventually incorporated regular exercise. When Sandra and I met, she was ready to begin her new fitness journey and as her personal trainer, I was able to guide her and help her reach her fitness goals. She brought focus, dedication and commitment to her new lifestyle, and made my job as her trainer an inspiring experience.

Her dedication and commitment to her health allowed her to go from weighing over 200 pounds to currently weighing 154 pounds. In November 2010, she ran her first 5k run and continues to set new fitness goals.

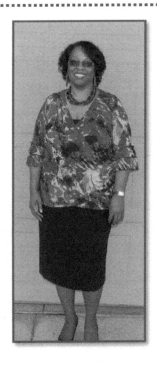

Before - April 2009, 219 lbs

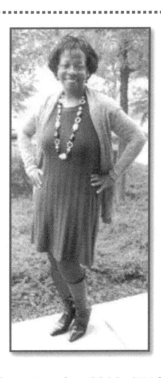

After - October 2010, 154 lbs

Sandra recently celebrated her forty-ninth birthday and her new life is the best present she could have given herself. Every time I see her, I am inspired by her transformation and honored to be a part of her fitness journey.

Just like Sandra, you too can reach your fitness goals. Embrace your age and view it as an asset and not a liability. Your age won't stop you from reaching your goals, but a lack of commitment and follow-through will. I have no doubt in my mind that you can do this. I am right here to guide you step-by-step.

If your age is preventing you from moving forward, refuse to be held hostage by a number.

Are you ready to unlock your fit?

Prepare to Succeed

Getting fit at any age can be a challenge, but planning for your fitness success can assist you in reaching your desired destination. Let me show you how to get on board and stay on board with your fitness goals at an older age.

- Make a list of challenges that are keeping you from setting and reaching your fitness/health goals. Be honest and make realistic goals to change these behaviors. Any behavior done consistently for more than thirty days can normally become a habit. Take one-step at a time to change these behaviors; be patient - change will not occur over night.

- Surround yourself with other women in your age group who are dedicated to getting fit. Forming a strong support system is essential to your success and will provide you with support from other women who may experience the same emotional and physical challenges.

If your age is preventing you from moving forward, refuse to be held hostage by a number and set realistic fitness goals for yourself.

- As you reach your goals, reward yourself with non-food items to celebrate your success. Possibly get a new dress, shoes or purse. Make it special to your likings.

- Share your accomplishments with individuals in your support system who love and believe in you. They won't downplay your success and they will know how hard you have worked to get there.

- Continue to hold yourself accountable to making progress and don't allow your age to be a barrier to reaching your fitness goals. In order to do this, find an accountability partner to help you stay consistent and dedicated. If you find yourself discouraged, address the causes of your discouragement and move forward.

- If you fall off track, do not beat yourself up. Get back up, brush the dust off and move forward with your fitness goals. Everyone gets side tracked every now and then.

- If you become bored with your fitness goals, set new ones. This will keep you engaged and excited about your fitness program and reaching your desired fitness destination.

- Take your workouts to the pool. As we age, we may experience arthritis and other joint problems. If you experience joint problems with physical activities, take your exercise to the pool. Exercising in the water places less stress on the joints and allows more pain-free movements.

Are You Afraid of What They May Say?

Let me ask you a few questions.

Have you allowed your unhealthy social environment affect your health? Do you struggle with saying no to your friends when they ask you out to fast food restaurants? How many times have your girlfriends talked you out of a workout to go shopping for a new pair of shoes?

If this is you, it is essential to remember that your environment can either help or hinder your progress towards getting healthier.

If you have thought about taking control of your environment but you've been afraid of what your friends and family may say, today is the day to speak up. It's time to finally talk with them and discuss your decision to get healthy.

During your discussion, express your need for support. You can express your need for support by painting a clear picture of what being supported looks like to you. By doing this, you are taking ownership of your decision to get healthy and allowing the people in your life to provide you with the support you need and desire. If you do not receive the encouragement and support you need, don't get discouraged. There are individuals out there who will support you on your fitness journey.

You can find this support by attending your local gym or wellness center where you will find other health-conscience people. In addition to attending your local gym and wellness center, the worldwide web provides numerous internet fitness groups to join for support, education and inspiration.

You may feel alone without the support of those close to you, but don't allow this to deter you from your commitment to your health. Change is a process for those in your life, therefore give them time and space to accept the changes you are making. Continue to remain committed to your health, and possibly your healthy changes may inspire those in your life to make healthy changes for themselves.

Below is a listing of community fitness sites. Use these chosen sites as well as discover your own on the World Wide Web.

If you are a member of a church, community organization or company, it is possible that you may want to create your own fitness support group.

Community Fitness Sites

www.sparkpeople.com

www.inspire.com

www.sweat365.com

www.fitness.com

It takes a village to get fit, therefore find a village that will support and encourage you on your fitness journey.

Chapter

There's an athlete in every woman dying to perform her best!

3

Unlock Your Fit

You're Not a Number

With so many pressures to be thin, many women feel the need to constantly weigh themselves and use the number on the scale as a baseline of their self-worth and level of attractiveness. In many ways, this is counterproductive.

Therefore, I need to take a moment to be honest with you. My honesty may break your heart, but I am here to guide you on the right path.

Are you ready to hear what I have to say?

The weight scale isn't your friend. I know, these are hard words to hear, but they are the truth. The weight scale has a tendency to not tell you the truth and depending on what time of the day you talk to her, she may tell you something different from the day before.

I know you and the scale have been friends for years, but it's time to limit the time you spend together. Your relationship with her has the potential to be detrimental to your mind and body.

Therefore, instead of focusing on the weight scale for affirmation, pay attention to your energy levels, how you feel in your clothes, have you lost inches, do you sleep better? Can you get through your day without feeling tired? Besides you can't gain fat weight overnight. If you focus on eating healthy, monitoring your exercise and physical activity levels, you will continue to lose weight. Is it wrong to want to know your weight? No, but if you allow the numbers on the scale to dictate your self-worth and level of fitness, it's time to get rid of her!

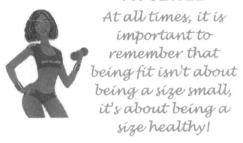

FIT JEWEL

At all times, it is important to remember that being fit isn't about being a size small, it's about being a size healthy!

Below you will discover ways to use the weight scale as a weight loss tool and not as a determining factor of the success of your fitness program and your self-worth.

Rules for Weighing Yourself

Weigh yourself in the morning before you have anything to drink or eat: Having fluid and food in the body will cause you to weigh more. For most women, this is very discouraging and can cause them to abandon their fitness program. Therefore when you weigh yourself, it is important to weigh early in the mornings prior to eating or drinking. The number on the scale at this time is your true weight.

Weigh yourself the same time every day: Your body weight fluctuates throughout the day. Therefore if you weigh yourself at 6am, choose this hour every time you weigh yourself in order to get a consistent weighing.

Do not weigh yourself every day: You cannot gain fat weight overnight. Your body will change weight on a daily basis based on hydration, hormonal and food levels. If you are menstruating, your body retains more fluid which will result in weight gain in the form of water. Weighing yourself everyday can become distracting and discouraging. It takes time to lose weight, be patient.

You're more than fat weight: Our body weight is composed of water, lean muscle tissue and fat. When you see a number on the scale, it doesn't tell you how much weight is in water, lean muscle tissue and fat. Therefore, don't get fixated with the number on the scale. For an example, I weigh 152 lbs and 113 lbs is composed of lean muscle tissue.

A Heart Beat Away

Unlocking your fit means more than just getting toned arms and a flat stomach. It also means discovering health issues that affect you as a woman.

Having a six...okay, a four pack and toned arms is a great reason to want to get in shape, but I challenge you to look for additional reasons. Make the decision to incorporate regular exercise, healthy eating into your life in order to help prevent the number one killer of women—heart disease. Let's talk about why it is so important to keep the heart healthy.

Why is your heart health more important than a six-pack?

The heart is the body's main engine that provides oxygen-rich blood to all functioning organs, tissues and bones. Making unhealthy lifestyle choices can increase your risk for heart disease and other lifestyle-related illnesses such as hypertension and diabetes. According to the American Heart Association, heart disease is the number one killer of women and every second a woman dies from heart disease, leaving behind many loved ones.

One major concern regarding heart disease is that many women have heart disease and don't know they have it. Just like hypertension (high blood pressure) heart disease can be a silent killer. Therefore, it is imperative that your health becomes a primary focal point in your life.

At the beginning of this fitness journey, your main concern for getting in shape may have been just to look great. As I mentioned before, looking great is a benefit of living a healthy life, but it should not be the driving force behind your decision to get in shape.

Are you aware of your heart's condition?

When was the last time you had a physical?

I understand how demanding life becomes. You have many roles and responsibilities, but your role needs to include being your own best friend. A best friend is honest, dependable, takes care of you and is loving.

Are you being all those things to yourself?

If you aren't being a best friend to yourself, it is time to start. The first step in becoming your best friend is to schedule an annual visit to the doctors to have your heart, cholesterol, blood pressure and triglycerides checked. Knowing your numbers (cholesterol, blood pressure) and family health history can help prevent you from becoming another statistic of heart disease.

The next step is to commit to some form of exercise or physical activity most days of the week. This can include a 10-15 minute walk during work, gardening, Zumba or riding your bike. It doesn't matter what exercise or physical activities you choose, just move your body. Your heart and waistline will say thank you.

It is important to remember that heart disease displays itself differently in women as compared to men. Therefore, become heart healthy and learn the signs and symptoms of heart disease. In addition to becoming heart healthy, become your sister's keeper and share this information with your girlfriends, sisters and mothers.

What are risk factors and symptoms of a heart attack/heart disease?

How can you avoid becoming another statistic of heart disease? You can accomplish this by recognizing the risk factors and symptoms of heart disease and heart attacks.

Risk Factors

Risk factors are conditions that place you at a higher chance for developing heart disease. They include smoking, a sedentary (non-active) life-style, obesity, family history of heart disease, hypertension, age, race and diabetes.

Although we cannot control age, race and family history, we can control the remaining risk factors. Scheduling regular physicals and blood work will keep you updated on your heart health. Do not be afraid to discuss health concerns with your doctor(s); they are there to provide you with guidance and information. Locate websites that provide you with current information on heart disease awareness and prevention.

Symptoms of Heart Disease

Symptoms of heart disease include but are not limited to nausea, back pain, shortness of breath, pain down the left side of the arm and chest pain (angina). If you experience any of these symptoms, seek medical attention.

Education and Awareness

The American Red Cross (ARC) has done an outstanding job with campaign RED. Campaign Red is an educational and awareness program dedicated to the education and prevention of heart disease in women. To learn more about heart disease and how to prevent it, log onto to www.goredforwomen.org.

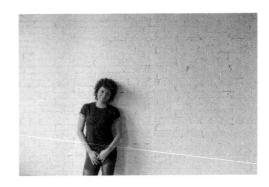

Heart Disease Statistics

Education + Knowledge= Empowerment

- African American women are at a greater risk for heart disease than Caucasian women.

- Nearly half (49 percent) of African American women have some form of heart disease.

- High blood pressure is considered a leading cause of heart disease and stroke.

- Heart disease is the number one killer and stroke is the number three killer of women over age 25.

- More women than men die each year from stroke. In 2004, more than 91,000 women died from stroke.

- Heart disease and stroke are the greatest health threat to women of varied ethnic backgrounds. Studies have shown only 21 percent of women realize they have heart disease.

- One in three adult women living in the USA has some form of cardiovascular disease (CVD).

- 58% of Caucasian women, 80% of African-American women, and 74% Hispanic-American women are overweight or obese.

- Women with diabetes are 2.5 times more likely to have heart attacks.

- 50% of Caucasian women, 64% of African-American women, 60% of Hispanic women, and 53% of Asian/Pacific Islander women are sedentary and get no leisure time physical activity.

Tips To Avoid Heart Disease

- Exercise regularly.
- Quit smoking.
- Maintain a healthy BMI (Body Mass Index) 18.5-24.9.
- Know your family health history of heart disease.

- Get regular cholesterol and blood lipid screenings.
- Stay away from saturated fats (fried foods) and foods high in sodium.
- Don't be afraid to ask your doctor questions about heart disease.
- Educate yourself about heart disease and be aware of the signs and symptoms.

Do you know your numbers? If you don't, make an appointment with your physician today. Your heart can't wait any longer.

Total Cholesterol: <200 mg/dL
LDL "Bad" Cholesterol:
Optimal: <100 mg/dL
Near optimal/Above Optimal: 100-129 mg/dL
Borderline High: 130-159 mg/dL
High: 160-189 mg/dL
Very High: 190 mg/dL and above
HDL ("Good") Cholesterol: 50 mg/dL or higher
Triglycerides: <150 mg/dL
Blood Pressure: <120/80 mmHg
Fasting Glucose: <100 mg/dL
Body Mass Index: <25
Waist Circumference: <35 inches

For more information on women and heart disease log on to the following websites.

American Heart Association

www.americanheart.org

National Heart, Lung & Blood Institute

www.nhlbi.nih.gov

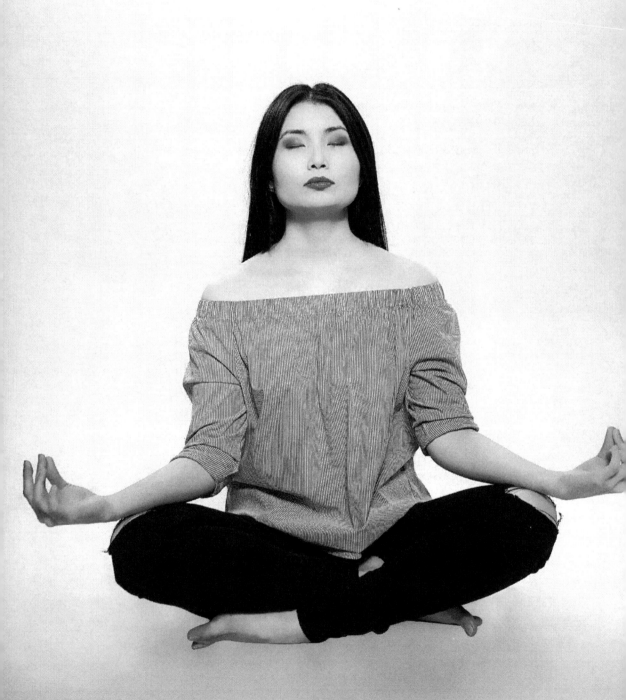

Chapter

You will become your thoughts, therefore choose them wisely!

4

**Change Your Mind,
Change Your Body**

How's Your Thought Life?

The current state of your body or health may be a direct reflection of your thought patterns about yourself and how you view your body and healthy living. Do you look at your body and speak negative words? Do you cringe at the thought of exercise and healthy eating?

If this is you, realize your thoughts can lead you down the road of fitness and weight loss success or your thoughts can lead you down the dead end road of overweight and unhappy.

Which road will you choose?

Think Success

Once I made the decision to become a professional fitness competitor, I realized how important my thoughts would be to the success of my career. The physical demands of training, injuries, the cost of competing, the struggle of being a full-time student and employee could have hindered me from reaching my goals if I allowed my thoughts to be thoughts of defeat. Therefore I realized early in my fitness career that my level of success heavily depended upon my thoughts. This truth holds the same for you and reaching your fitness goals.

During moments of physical and mental fatigue, I would speak words of affirmation to myself. When negative thoughts crossed my mind, I would quickly replace them with positive ones. On this fitness journey, you will have to create your own positive thoughts to help you reach your destination.

Maybe you have called yourself negative names or maybe you have told yourself that you will never get the weight off because you have tried everything in the past. Today is new experience and in order to be successful you will have to change your negative thought patterns.

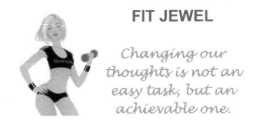

FIT JEWEL

Changing our thoughts is not an easy task, but an achievable one.

What have you been saying to yourself?

Take Control of Your Thoughts

In order to create positive thoughts that would assist me in reaching my goals, I created my three D's of fitness success. The three D's of success created a road map for thinking that allowed me to challenge my thought life and accomplish many of my goals.

I want to share my three D's of success with you. Use my three D's or create your own.

 1   **The First D Is For Desire.**

What do you desire?

- Do you desire to be able to run and play with your children without getting tired?
- To run a marathon?
- Look at yourself in the mirror unclothed and like what you see?
- Be more intimate with your husband and feel great about yourself?
- Get off blood pressure medication?

Whatever you desire, it has to be motivating enough to cause you to create and take the necessary steps to reach your destination. Desire has to be internal and it is something that doesn't have to be explained to anyone. Your desire has to be great enough to provoke a change within yourself and no one else.

2 The Second D Is For Discipline.

Many of us do not like the word discipline, as it conveys hard work. Discipline is something you must possess in order to reach your desired goal. It may mean getting up an hour earlier to get to the gym, or it could mean telling your closest friends you can't hang out all night because you need eight hours of sleep to have an effective fitness training session the next day. If you lack discipline, it will be hard to reach your fitness destination.

Ask yourself if you are willing to practice discipline on a consistent basis in order to reach your desired goal. The answer to this question will help you determine your current level of commitment to your fitness-training program.

3 The Last D Stands For Determination.

Determination is something I hold very dear to my heart. There have been many times in life where chaos has threatened to take control. During these moments, I had to make the choice to stay determined to reach my goals. It is essential to remember that chaos in your life does not constitute a reason to stop working towards your goals. Make the choice to work around your obstacles and refuse to accept "NO" for an answer. Do you have a desire?

Are you disciplined enough to reach that desire?

Are you determined to move forward when life gets tough?

If you are currently finding it difficult to reach your fitness goals, the tips below will provide you with a starting point. Need support? Don't be afraid to ask for it.

Get On Board with Your Dreams

- Refuse to accept negative thoughts from yourself or other people. You can't stop every thought from coming into your mind, but you can block many of them.

- Write down your goals and the steps required to reach them. Having a visual reference can help you get excited about your goals. Create a vision board and place it somewhere visible.

- Only share your dreams with people who believe in you and want to support you. Having negative people in your life is toxic and unproductive.

- Take daily steps to reach your destination. Don't get overwhelmed with the destination, instead focus on the process. By doing this, you will feel less pressure and stress to reach your goals.

- Be proud of the progress you are making, whether big or small. Don't wait until you reach your goal to celebrate. Every day that you move in a positive direction towards your goal is a day to be celebrated.

- Do not beat yourself up for not reaching your goal by the deadline you've set. It's not failure on our part, we may have just set unrealistic goals within an unrealistic period of time. When this happens, re-evaluate your goals and set more realistic ones in a more reasonable time frame.

Failure Is Not An Option

Setting fitness goals and following through is a challenge for many women. Whether it is work, family responsibilities or exhaustion, women often find themselves at the bottom of their workload and to do list.

We all have been there and some of us are still there - but here's the reality. You have to **TAKE** time for yourself in order to change your health, and by no means will this change be easy.

The journey of change will consist of many trials and tribulations, but will result in personal growth and development. There will be days when you want to throw in the towel and go back to old habits and negative ways of thinking. When these moments happen, say aloud, "Failure is not an option." Say it with authority and inner strength. When your support system is not as supportive as they once were, say it again, "Failure is not an option." With tears rolling down your face, pick your head up, put your shoulders back and say it again.

If change were easy, more people would invest the time and pain needed to become the person they really desire to become. I commend you for taking this journey and I am walking with you step-by-step cheering you on. Can you hear me yelling your name?

It takes courage and determination to change things you do not like about yourself, and on the days you are feeling lonely and believe no one understands what you are going through, know there are millions of other women who are struggling with the same issues you are. It is time to no longer accept nothing less but the best from yourself.

Are you ready to finally let go of all the excuses and fears? If you are, the world is anxiously waiting for the arrival of a new and improved you. Don't give up, you have come too far!

Step out and show them who you really are!

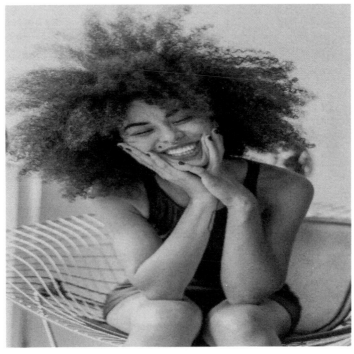

Chapter 5

Change can be a painful process, but it's worth the pain.

Ten Days of Inner Discovery

Seek and You Shall Find

The only items required for this section is a pen, open heart and mind. Before you begin journaling find a quiet place where you can process your thoughts and emotions without being interrupted. Being alone with yourself will provide you with the time needed in order to answer the following questions. As you move forward with this process, it is essential to understand that participating in Ten Days of Inner Discovery will require you to be honest with yourself about your past and the person you have become.

As you journal, I'd encourage you to be open about exploring areas within yourself that you may have been hidden away. Discovering answers to hard ask questions may lead you down a path of emotional healing and freedom. Often times our body image and self-esteem are a reflection of our past experiences and by acknowledging the pain from these past experiences we can potentially move forward in life.

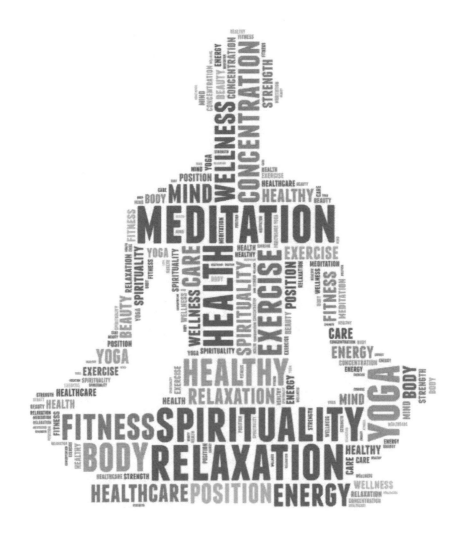

Day 1

Today, you are going to take 15-20 minutes to reflect over your childhood experiences and write about them. Can you recall certain defining moments in your childhood? Were these moments happy or sad? Many of our behaviors and attitudes including our body image are shaped from our childhood experiences.

Take your time and don't be afraid to dive deep into your past.

Day 1 Journal Entry	Date:

Day 2: External Exploration

Write down all the physical things you do not like about yourself. Yes, I said that correctly - we are going to write down all the physical things we do not like about ourselves. You probably have a puzzled look on your face. Stay with me; by the end of Day 10 you will understand completely.

Day 2 Journal Entry	Date:

Day 3: Mirror, Mirror on the Wall

Write down all the things you love about yourself. This task will be difficult for some and easy for others. If in your past people criticized you and told you that you were worthless, then you may have a hard time finding the good things within. However, dig deep and write down at least five things you love about yourself.

**Day 3
Journal Entry**

Date:

Day 4: Internal Revelation

Today's assignment is going to be thought-provoking. Make sure you have at least 15-20 minutes to write in your journal. Answer the following questions.

Day 4 Journal Entry

Date:

1. Are you an honest and trust worthy person?

2. When you give someone your word, do you follow through?

3. Do you value family and friends?

4. Are you self-centered and insensitive to others feelings?

5. Are you truly happy with your life?

6. Are past hurts keeping you from moving forward?

7. Do you believe life has a great plan for you?

8. Do you look at other people's lives and envy them?

9. Do you believe you can accomplish whatever you put your mind to?

10. Do you try new things or are you stuck in a rut?

11. Is your self-worth based on other people's opinion of you?

12. Do you seek happiness in money or material things?

Day 5: Today Is Dedicated To Pure Relaxation

Find a special place where no one else is allowed. Burn an aromatherapy candle, play some soft music and set the lights dimly. It may sound like you are preparing a place for a romantic dinner with someone else, but you are actually preparing for a special moment with yourself. Take 15 minutes to pray or meditate on your day. Do not feel bad; the earth will continue to rotate without you being there to turn it on its axis. **Health Tip:** Meditation and relaxation have been shown to improve blood pressure and overall health.Therefore incorporate at least 5-10 minutes per day for meditation. You're worth it.

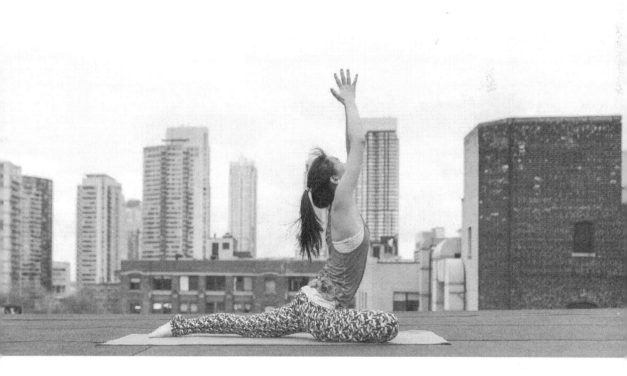

Day 6: Write Your Vision

Write down your short-term (4-6 months) and long-term (1 year or longer) fitness goals and create a plan of action needed to reach these goals. Get descriptive and provide measurable means to track your progress.

**Day 6
Journal Entry**

Date:

Short Term Goals:

Long Term Goals:

Day 7: Have a night out on the town

Today you are going to make plans to have a "Girl's Night Out." This is not a suggestion, it is an order. Blow the dust off your heels, call up a few of your friends and plan a great night out. On this night out, do not talk about your beautiful kids, job or wonderful spouse.

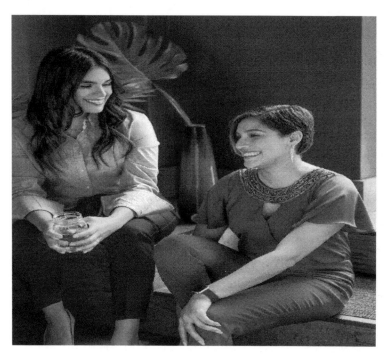

Day 8: Break Free

Today we are going to make plans to adventure somewhere new. I do not know about you, but sometimes I feel stuck in a rut and need to get out of it. Traveling the same route to work every day, doing the same tasks at work and going through the routine of a normal day can get boring.

Do you ever feel this way?

When was the last time you took a different route to work?

What about the last time you went to your favorite restaurant--
did you order the same meal?

Break free and do something unusual today.

Day 9: Ready for Change

Today we are going to reflect on Days 1-8. Be honest with yourself about what you have discovered regarding your personality, self-image, childhood experiences, dreams and goals.

Decide whether you are at a point in your life where you can commit to making a change. Take time; do not rush through this process.

If you cannot take the first step by yourself, find someone you trust to help you move forward. I have learned it is great to have support when we are going through tough moments in life.

Day 9 Journal Entry	Date:
Honest Reflection: Write about your discovery	

Day 10: New Beginning

Today is a celebration of a new life! Old behaviors, negative attitudes and negative thought patterns are kicked out the door. No longer will you allow other people to define who you are and you are working on changing any negative behaviors you have discovered. You will no longer base your happiness on your clothing size or the numbers on the scale. You are empowered by taking time to love and care for your body. It is a new day and a newer you. Take what you have learned over these 10 days and continue to work on who you want to become from a mental, emotional, spiritual and physical standpoint.

Continual Quest

It is essential to remember that when it comes to self-discovery, there is no plateau. The search for meaning and purpose is a continuum throughout our lives and if we ever decide to stop searching, our growth will become stagnant and we will lose the desire to thrive. Throughout this growth process, continue to set new and challenging fitness and personal goals for yourself. Smile more often and don't be afraid to look in the mirror at the real you. The stage lights are off and it is safe to remove the mask for good. The new you is more confident, fit, empowered and ready to take on the world one day at a time.

A Never Ending Covenant

As you continue on this quest, I want you to make a vow of commitment to yourself. Taking a vow of commitment to yourself will keep you striving every day to live up to the promises you have made to yourself.

When we get married, we give vows to our future spouse. We speak these vows in front of God, friends and family and try to uphold every one of them - so why can't we make vows to ourselves and uphold them?

FIT JEWEL

If we can make and try to keep vows to our spouse, why not make vows to ourselves?

You can use the vows below that I have written to myself, or write your own. Once you have written your vows, display them in a place where you can see them on a daily basis. You can place them on your bathroom mirror or your refrigerator or at the office - it's your choice, just make sure they are visible.

On the days you are not feeling great about yourself, you will have a written reminder of your greatness. Rehearse them in your mind and bind them around your heart by carefully pondering and applying them to your daily life. Greatness is in you, do you believe it?

My Vows

1   I will always love and respect myself.

I will laugh at myself when I make mistakes.   2

3   I will never settle for less than my worth.

I will love myself when others have forsaken me.   4

5   I will always be honest with myself.

I will push myself when others say I cannot make it.   6

7   I will not look at my past and allow it to define my future.

I will be my best friend, biggest fan and greatest encourager.   8

9   I will not allow the world's standard of beauty to define me.

I will not be defined by what I do, my body or my bank account   10

Chapter

The truth of who you are will never be discovered in front of a mirror.

6

Honest Reflection

Refuse the Norm

Continue to discover the qualities that define you that go beyond your physical appearance.

Take a moment to answer the following questions.

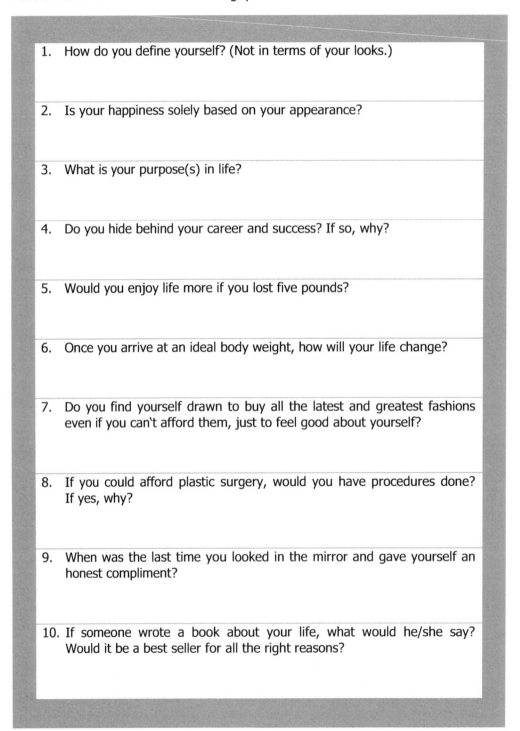

1. How do you define yourself? (Not in terms of your looks.)

2. Is your happiness solely based on your appearance?

3. What is your purpose(s) in life?

4. Do you hide behind your career and success? If so, why?

5. Would you enjoy life more if you lost five pounds?

6. Once you arrive at an ideal body weight, how will your life change?

7. Do you find yourself drawn to buy all the latest and greatest fashions even if you can't afford them, just to feel good about yourself?

8. If you could afford plastic surgery, would you have procedures done? If yes, why?

9. When was the last time you looked in the mirror and gave yourself an honest compliment?

10. If someone wrote a book about your life, what would he/she say? Would it be a best seller for all the right reasons?

Part II

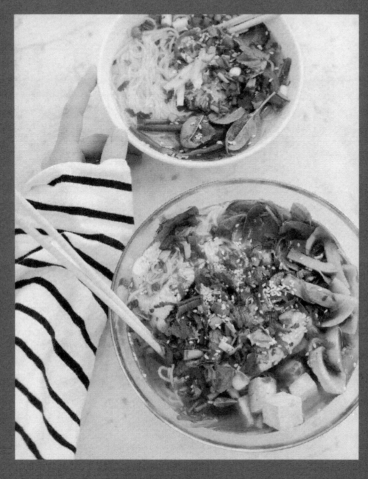

Fuel Your Success

C h a p t e r

Diets don't work, lifestyle changes do!

7

No More Dieting

No More Dieting

Creating a healthy perspective of yourself was the first step on your fitness journey. The next step is to learn how to provide your body with healthy nourishment in order to reach a healthy body weight and remain fit for life.

This section won't teach you how to diet. Diets are often depriving, costly and don't result in permanent weight loss. Therefore, in this chapter you will learn the importance of macro-nutrients, identify their function in your body, discover how to eat healthy well-balanced meals and learn how to make healthy behavior changes that will ultimately lead to making better food choices and permanent weight loss.

Besides, how many diets have you tried with the hopes of losing weight only to find yourself hungry, deprived and pounds heavier? Dieting is over, it's time for you to make a lifestyle change.

I understand how changing your lifestyle and behaviors can be a hard concept to accept due to the fact that the diet and fitness industry comes up with a new diet every other day of the week that promises drastic weight loss with only the popping of a few pills and only 3-minutes of exercise a day, but I need you to ask yourself a question. If losing weight were that simple wouldn't everyone in America be at a healthy weight?

The truth is, one of the only ways to reach permanent weight loss is to provide the body with proper balanced nutrition in moderation, exercise on a regular basis and changing your lifestyle.

FIT JEWEL

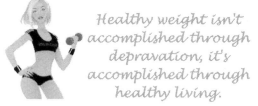

Healthy weight isn't accomplished through depravation, it's accomplished through healthy living.

If you are, then it's time to learn the importance of healthy eating.

Why Most Diets Don't Work

Most diets are restrictive: Restricting certain foods groups from your nutritional plan may cause your body to miss out on essential nutrients. Restricting these essential nutrients may cause certain health problems if absent from your diet for too long.

Most diets severely decrease your caloric intake: The body requires a certain amount of calories to perform the basic functions of life such as breathing and digestion. Consuming low amounts of calories can cause your body to use other sources such as your muscle tissue (protein) for energy. Very low calories diets can ultimately disrupt your metabolism. In the long run, this may actually make it harder to burn calories and lose weight.

Diets are unrealistic and difficult to follow: Choosing to stay on a diet for an extended amount of time is unrealistic. With low amounts of food intake and restriction, diets are often short lived and lead to additional weight gain. You can't eat grapefruit for the rest of your life.

Diets have regimented meal plans: Regimented diets often require the dieter to either buy expensive diet shakes or meals, or stock up their fridge with very specific regimented foods. This can be costly and boring to the palate, leaving you wanting foods higher in calories and flavor.

Most diets make you dependent on prepackaged meals: Most diet plans require you to purchase their foods products as a tool for weight loss. In the long run, this can hinder you from learning how to cook, prepare and determine proper portion sizes of food. No one can remain on diet products forever, and eventually you have to learn how to eat in the real world.

Chapter

Consuming more protein will not cause you to grow bulky muscles!

8

Protein: The Building Blocks

Macro-Fit

Although there are many nutrients that are important to your health, three nutrients make up the majority of your nutritional requirements. These nutrients are termed "macro-nutrients" and consist of protein, carbohydrates and fats. When consumed in balance, macro-nutrients can provide your body with the proper nutrition for the growth and repair of your body's tissues.

For many women attempting to get in shape, there is a great amount of confusion surrounding the roles of these macros - especially protein. Therefore, we will first discuss the role of protein, how much is required for your body and what role it plays in getting fit.

Protein: The Building Blocks

Protein is one of the most popular macros. Everywhere you turn - whether it's in a women's health or fitness magazine - there's talk about the latest and greatest sources of protein. But for some women, they have been led to believe if they consume protein that they will gain too much muscle and look manly.

This is a myth, and although protein is required for muscle growth and repair, it has many other functions in the body and consuming protein alone will not cause your muscles to grow manly.

Before I go any further, I promise I'm not going to give you a chemistry lesson on protein, but I will provide you with basic essential information.

What's the truth about protein?

Protein is the major functional and structural component of all cells in the body. Everything from skin, hair, nails, enzymes and collagen are formed from individual proteins (amino acids). If consumed in inadequate amounts, you risk hair loss, skin problems, stunted

muscle growth and many other health-related issues. To keep it basic, protein is needed in your everyday life for all body functions, including repairing your toned muscles from resistance-training and exercise.

In order to clarify some of the confusion on protein, below you will find frequently asked questions accompanied with the answers regarding the role of protein in regards to getting fit.

FAQS Regarding Protein

Q.

HOW MUCH PROTEIN DO I REALLY NEED?

A.

The amount of protein you consume is based on your current lifestyle, age, sex and fitness goals. If you are a sedentary person (inactive), your requirements are lower versus the requirements of someone more active who resistance trains.

For those women who aren't as active, it is recommended that you consume at least 0.8 grams of protein per kilogram of body weight per day.

For more active women who resistance train and desire to build lean muscle, your intake will be higher. For optimal recovery, consume at least 1.0 gram of protein per kilogram of body weight.

No worries, I will show you how to determine your body weight in kilograms.

Use the following equation to determine these samples of protein intake. (See below)

Protein Equation:
Plug in your body weight

Example: If you weigh 150 pounds and are inactive (sedentary)

1. Divide your body weight by 2.2. This will convert pounds into kilograms (150/2.2)= 68 kilograms

2. Multiply 68 kilograms by 0.8 (68x 0.8)= 54

3. Consume approximately 54 grams of protein per day

Q.

HOW CAN I ADD PROTEIN TO MY DIET?

A.

Protein can be found in foods such as beans, nuts, eggs, dairy products, fish, bison, lean beef and seafood. When choosing meat, look for sources that are low in amounts of saturated fat*. If you are often on-the-go, purchasing a protein powder and a shaker bottle can provide you with a quick and easy way to get optimal consumption of protein. Just add 1-2 scoops of protein based on the grams per serving, add water, shake and go.

* Saturated fat content is generally located on the nutrition label of the package. Look for items that have less than 5% of the Daily Value (DV) from saturated fat*

Q.

I'M VEGAN, HOW CAN I GET PROTEIN?

A.

You can get your required protein intake by consuming a variety of grains, beans, legumes, soy, tofu, veggie burgers and nuts. The key to your protein consumption is to consume a variety and combination of these food items.

Q.

WHAT ARE ESSENTIAL AND NON-ESSENTIAL AMINO ACIDS?

A.

There are 20 amino acids needed for proper functioning of the human body. Of these 20 amino acids, 8 are considered essential. Essential means the body does not produce them, therefore they must be consumed in the diet. The other 12 amino acids are non-essential, which means the body naturally produces them. To find out more information on amino acids visit www.webmd.com.

Q.

WHAT IS THE BEST FORM OF PROTEIN POWDER?

A.

There are many forms of protein powder, but whey protein has one of the highest biological values (BV). Biological value is defined by the amount of protein that is readily available and used by the body. You can find whey protein in many nutrition and health food stores.

In order to find a whey protein that works for you, experiment with different brands and flavors. Whey protein is a by-product of milk, therefore if you are lactose intolerant, this may not work well with your digestive system. If this is the case, you may want to use soy protein or find a whey product that has reduced lactose or is lactose free.

A.

A complete protein is a protein that contains all 20 amino acids needed for the body to function properly. Most animal products are sources of complete proteins, whereas plant proteins do not contain all essential amino acids.

A.

Yes. It is important to replenish the body with protein (amino acids) after a training session. Consuming protein within 30-45 minutes after a workout is important for muscle tissue repair and recovery. After your workout, consume at least 25 grams of protein with a fast absorbing carbohydrate (sports drink such as Gatorade™, PowerAde™, or fruit). Some studies believe combining protein and a fast absorbing carbohydrate will transport amino acids into the cells at a faster rate. Faster delivery equals faster recovery.

A.

Purchasing RTD's (Ready-To-Drink) (which are pre-packaged protein drinks) is a quick and convenient way to meet your protein needs. RTD's come in various brands and flavors. These drinks may be pricey, but are convenient.

Before purchasing, read ingredient and nutrition labels. Reading these labels will help you determine the amount of calories, carbohydrates, protein and fat per serving in each drink. Some of these drinks are high in calories and sugar so read ALL labels.

Another convenient way to consume protein is to purchase a tub of protein powder along with a shaker bottle. You can purchase snacks bags and measure out the required amount per serving and place in your gym or lunch bag. The only thing required to make a protein shake is water and a shaker bottle. Shake, enjoy and go!

A.

No. Consuming more protein will not get you in better shape at a faster rate. A combination of resistance training, regular cardiovascular activities and healthy eating is required to reach optimal health and fitness levels. Protein is used to help build and repair damaged tissue, but consumption alone will not get you to your desired fitness level faster.

A.

No. Building bulky muscles should not be a concern for the average woman. Genetics, sex related hormones (testosterone) and heavy resistance training (weight lifting) are the main factors in building bulky muscle. Consuming the appropriate amount of protein in conjunction with light resistance training will aid you in building lean, toned muscles.

Protein Sources

Chicken	Edamame (soybeans)
Beans	Egg whites
Tofu	Lean Beef (93%)
Nuts and Seeds	Fish (Salmon, Halibut, Tilapia)
Peanut Butter	Ground Turkey
Buffalo	Cottage Cheese
Venison	Almond Butter

Additional Protein Sources

Fish

Tilapia	**Whiting**
4 oz 100 kcal	4 oz 77 kcal
2.5g fat	2g fat
20g protein	18g protein
Cod	**Flounder**
4 oz 80 kcal	40z 120 kcal
3g fat	6g fat
14g protein	17g protein
Wild Alaskan Salmon	**Canned Tuna**
4 oz 80 kcal	(In water or olive oil)
1.5g fat	5 oz 50 kcal
16g protein	1g fat
	11g protein

Deli Meats (low sodium)

Turkey Breasts	**Roast Beef**
6 slices 50 kcal	6 slices 50 kcal
1g fat	2g fat
8g protein	10g protein
Ham	**Chicken Breasts**
6 slices 50 kcal	6 slices 50 kcal
1g fat	1g fat
9g protein	9g protein

Chicken

Chicken Breast
4 oz 120 kcal
22g fat
19g protein

Ground Chicken
4 oz 180 kcal
11gfat
19g protein

Beef

Lean ground beef 93%
4 oz 180 kcal
8g fat
24g protein

Turkey

Turkey breast cutlets
4 oz 120 kcal
0.5g fat
28gprotein

Turkey Bacon (low sodium)
1 slice 35 kcal
3g fat
2g protein

Ground Turkey
4 oz 140 kcal
3.5g fat
27g protein

Turkey Sausage
2 oz 100 kcal
5g fat
8g protein

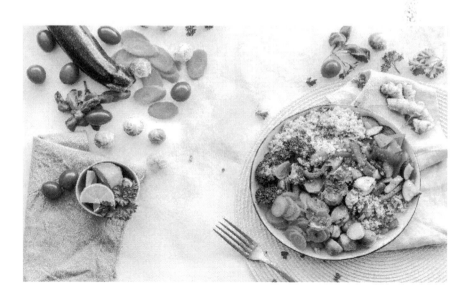

Chapter

Consuming healthy dietary fat doesn't make you gain weight, consuming the wrong calories and too many of them will make you gain weight.

9

Fat Attack

Fat Attack

The second macro-nutrient we will discuss is dietary fat. Over the years, dietary fat has earned a negative reputation based on increased health issues related to high consumptions of saturated and trans fats in most American's diets. Saturated and trans fats have been linked to alarming rates of obesity, heart disease and other health related issues, but all fats are not created equal and dietary fat isn't to be solely blamed for the increasing rates of obesity in America.

Yes, believe it or not, there are good sources of dietary fat and it is important to understand that almost all foods have some form of fat, but the fats you want as a part of your regular nutritional plan are unsaturated fats, which include monounsaturated and polyunsaturated fat. These fats when eaten in moderation are known to provide the body with many health benefits such as lowering your bad cholesterol(LDL), increasing your good cholesterol (HDL), and fighting inflammation.

The Department of Health and Human Services (H.H.S.) recommends no more than 20 to 35 percent of your diet come from fat. This means that the majority of your dietary fat should come from unsaturated fat, which includes monounsaturated and polyunsaturated fat.

The Good, Bad and the Ugly

Understanding the difference between healthy and unhealthy fats is important in order to make healthier food choices for you and your family. Therefore, let's discuss the four major categories of dietary fat which include, unsaturated fat, trans fat, monounsaturated fats and polyunsaturated fats.

Unsaturated fats (which include monounsaturated and polyunsaturated fats) are considered healthy sources of fat which have been shown to help lower your risk of heart disease by lowering your bad cholesterol (low-density lipoprotein) (LDL) and increasing your good cholesterol high-density lipoproteins (HDL). Unsaturated fats are found in foods such as nuts, seeds, olive oil and peanut butter.

One polyunsaturated fat known to be beneficial to your health is Omega-3 Fatty Acids. Studies have shown that Omegas 3's appear to decrease your risk of Coronary Artery Disease (C.A.D.) and may protect against irregular heartbeats and help lower blood pressure levels.

Now that we have discussed the categories of healthy fat (good fat), let's discuss the two categories of unhealthy fats (bad fats). The two categories include, saturated fats and trans fats. These fats have been linked to causing heart disease, diabetes and other major health concerns. Food sources that contain saturated and trans fats include baked goods, cakes, pies, red meat cheese and diary. It is recommended that you eat these foods sparingly due to the health concerns linked to their consumption.

Can you avoid dietary fat? No, and neither should you try. Instead of completely removing dietary fat from your meals, focus on consuming healthy sources of fat found in products such as nuts, fresh water fish, peanut butter (in moderation), nuts, seeds, olive oil and avocados.

It is also important to understand that although good sources of fat are needed in your nutritional plan, when compared to other macro-nutrients, fat contains more calories per gram (9 calories per gram). Therefore, consume in moderation.

FAQS Regarding Fat

Below you will find answers to questions most frequently asked about dietary fat.

> ## Q.
> ### WHAT IS SATURATED FAT?

A.

Saturated fat is an unhealthy fat found in many foods such as meat, eggs, cheese, fried foods, crackers, cookies, desserts, whole milk, palm oil and coconut oil. Animal fats are the primary source of saturated fat and should be consumed in moderation.

The U.S.D.A. recommends that less than 10 percent of our total daily calories come from saturated fat. Consuming saturated fat on a regular basis can lead to coronary heart disease and other heart related ailments, therefore saturated fat should be consumed in small amounts.

> ## Q.
> ### WHAT ARE TRANS FATS?

A.

Trans fats are unhealthy fats used to preserve the shelf life of many products. trans fats can be found in fried foods, baked goods, chips, cookies and crackers. One common trans fat is partially hydrogenated oils which are used to keep the crunch in snacks like chips and crackers.

It is recommended that no more than 1% of your daily calories come from trans fats. To avoid consuming these fats, read ingredient labels and be aware that some products may list a product as "Trans Fat Free" if a single serving contains less than 0.5 grams. Always read the fine print.

> ## Q.
> ### HOW DO I DETERMINE HOW MUCH FAT TO CONSUME?

A.

1. Determine your total calorie intake for the day.

2. Multiply that number by .20 (lower intake of fat) or by .35 (higher intake of fat)

Example: (To figure out the amount of fat you would consume on a daily caloric diet of 2,000 calories: Multiply 2,000 by 0.20 or 0.35 and then divide that number by 9, **(9 equals the number of calories per gram of fat.)** Based on a 2,000 calorie-a-day diet, this amounts to between 44-78 grams.

Fat consumed based on 20%

2000 X .20 = 400
400/9 = 44 grams

Fat consumed based on 35%

2000 X .35 = 700
700/9 = 78 grams

> ## Q.
> ### WHAT ARE MONO AND POLYUNSATURATED FATS?

A.

Mono and polyunsaturated fats are healthy fats that yield many health benefits when consumed. Foods such as olive oil, fish, seeds, peanut butter and nuts are great sources of healthy fats.

One particularly good fat is Omega-3 fatty acids. Studies have shown that Omega-3 fatty acids have the ability to protect the heart's vessels, prevent inflammation and some forms of Omega-3 are needed for brain, heart and eye health. The majority of your dietary fat should come from sources of mono or polyunsaturated fats.

Q.

HOW MUCH DIETARY FAT DO I NEED?

A.

It is recommended that no more than 20-35% of your total daily calories should come from fat and from mono and polyunsaturated sources.

Guidelines for Fat Consumption

Saturated Fat: less than 10%

Mono and Polyunsaturated: at least 20%

Trans Fat: no more than 1 percent

Samples of healthy daily allowances of fat consumption:

1,800 calories a day:

- 40 to 70 grams of total fat

- 14 grams or less of saturated fat

- 2 grams or less of Trans fat

2,200 calories a day:

- 49 to 86 grams of total fat

- 17 grams or less of saturated fat

- 3 grams or less of Trans fat

2,500 calories a day:

- 56 to 97 grams of total fat

- 20 grams or less of saturated fat

- 3 grams or less of Trans fat

Q.

HOW CAN I CUT BACK ON EATING BAD FATS?

A.

There are many ways to cut back on eating bad or unhealthy fats, which include:

- Remove skin from chicken, turkey and other poultry before cooking. Skin contains fat.

- When re-heating soups or stews, skim the solid fats from the top before serving.

- Drink low fat (1%) or fat-free (skim) milk rather than whole or 2% milk, or almond milk.

- Purchase low-fat or non-fat versions of your favorite cheese and other milk or dairy products.

- In order to satisfy your sweet tooth, reach for a low-fat or fat-free version of your favorite ice cream or frozen dessert. These versions usually contain less saturated fat, but be aware of sugar content in these food items. The removal of fat sometimes leads to adding additional sugar for taste.

- Use low fat margarine spreads instead of butter. Most margarine spreads contain less saturated fat than butter. Look for a spread that is low in saturated fat and does not contain trans fats.

- Choose baked goods, breads, and desserts that are low in saturated fat. You can find the fat content on the Nutrition Facts label.

- Pay attention at snack time. Some convenience snacks (such as sandwich crackers) contain saturated fat. Choose instead to have non-fat or low-fat yogurt, a piece of fruit or lightly salted nuts.

- Choose leaner cuts of meat that do not have a marbled appearance (where the fat appears embedded in the meat). Choose leaner cuts (including top round and sirloin) and trim all visible fat off meats before eating.

- Read all food labels and be conscious of what you are eating.

HEALTHY FAT		
Polyunsaturated Fats		
Vegetable Oils (Safflower, Corn, and Canola)		
Cold Water Fish (salmon, mackerel)		
Flaxseeds	Flax Oil	
Monounsaturated Fats		
Avocadoes	Peanuts	Almonds
Fish (Omega-3 fatty acids)	Olive Oil	Walnuts
Sunflower seeds	Peanut Butter	

UNHEALTHY FAT	
Saturated Fats	
Animal products such as meat, poultry, seafood, dairy products, lard, butter, coconut, palm, and other tropical oils.	
Trans Fats	
Partially hydrogenated vegetable oils, commercially-baked goods such as crackers, cookies and cakes, fried foods such as donuts, French fries, shortening and margarine.	

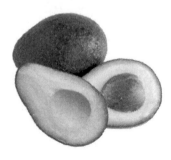

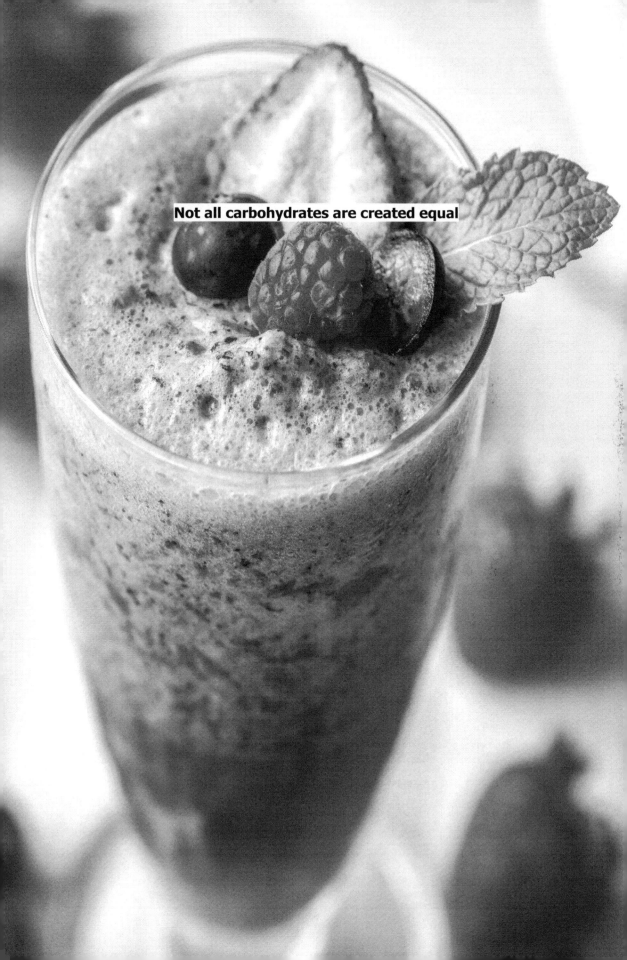

Not all carbohydrates are created equal

Chapter

Carbs are your friend, you just have to befriend the right ones!

10

Carbs: The Energy Makers

The Energy Maker

Carbohydrates, just like fat, have earned a negative reputation over the years due to increased health-related issues such as Type 2 Diabetes and Obesity. It has been proven that American's consume excessive amounts of sugar found in processed foods such as cakes, donuts, sugary energy drinks, coffee drinks, white breads and white pasta - which are all devoid of many healthy nutrients. But are all sugars bad for one's health and created equal? No, all sugars are not created equal, and there are healthy forms of sugars.

With so many rumors, are you afraid of consuming carbohydrates?

It is important to understand that although carbohydrates have been given a bad name, all carbohydrates aren't the culprit of poor health and weight gain. Poor health and weight gain are the combined result of limited physical activity, diets high in calories and unhealthy lifestyle behaviors. For years you may have stayed away from carbohydrates, not knowing the truth behind these important macro-nutrients. Therefore, let's paint a different picture and learn the truth about carbohydrates.

What Are Carbohydrates?

Carbohydrates are the body's main fuel source that provides energy for basic bodily functions such as breathing, body movements, digestion and normal heart functioning. When compared to fat and protein, carbohydrates are broken down at a quicker rate and are more readily available than any other macro-nutrient. For many reasons this is beneficial, but over the years there has been a great amount of dispute regarding whether or not a person should consume carbohydrates or stay away from them.

In the early 2000's, this dispute became profitable for many companies that focused on low-carb diet plans that encouraged low-to-no consumption of carbohydrates. This short-lived diet craze created the buzz that carbohydrates were the enemy within the food industry, but this picture wasn't painted as clear as it should have been.

Have ever been on an extremely low carbohydrate diet? if you have, you probably experienced low energy levels and restricted mental focus. If this occurred, it was a result of low glucose or blood sugar levels. As stated earlier, carbohydrates are an important source of fuel for the bodies basic functioning and without the proper amount of carbohydrates from the right sources, the body doesn't function at its best levels.

I understand with all the differing opinions on carbohydrates if you are still apprehensive about consuming carbohydrates, but I want to put your fears to rest and teach you more about carbohydrates.

FIT JEWEL

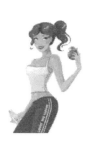

It is essential to understand that you don't have to completely avoid carbohydrates, rather learn which types to consume, how many grams per day and the right time of the day to utilize them.

Let's move on and learn more about the energy makers.

Why So Much Drama?

Right about now you might be a little confused about carbohydrates due to the fact that you have always heard carbohydrates are the enemy. Let me emphasize that carbohydrates aren't the enemy and there's no need for you to deal with the carbohydrate drama anymore.

First things first - let's identify the different types of carbohydrates.

There are two primary types of carbohydrates: they are complex carbohydrates (3 or more sugar molecules) and simple sugars (1 or 2 sugar molecules). Carbohydrates are categorized by the number of sugar molecules they are made of and each type of carbohydrate metabolizes differently in the body based on their chemical structure.

What are complex carbohydrates?

Complex carbohydrates are made up of 3 or more sugar molecules. This molecular structure results in a slower absorption rate into our blood stream as compared to simple sugars. This slow absorption process provides the body with sustained amounts of energy and you are less likely to experience the blood sugar spikes compared to consuming simple sugars. Therefore, it is recommended that the majority of your carbohydrates come from complex carbohydrate sources such as whole grain breads, sweet potatoes, quinoa, brown rice, steel cut oatmeal and vegetables. We have learned about complex carbohydrates, now let's learn about simple sugars.

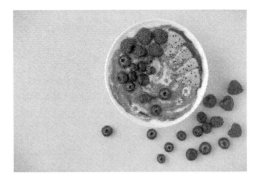

What are simple sugars?

Simple sugars are made up of 1 or 2 sugar molecules. Their molecular structure results in faster sugar absorption into our bodies and high spikes in blood glucose or blood sugar

levels. Consumption of simple sugars provides quick, but inadequate, amounts of sustained energy. These sugars are found in processed foods such as, baked goods, milk products, honey, corn syrup, molasses, brown sugar and maple syrup. Consuming high amounts of simple sugars has been linked to diabetes, weight gain and other health related issues including inflammation. Therefore, these should be consumed in moderation.

The Great Crash

Let's travel down memory lane for a moment.

Have you ever had one of those mornings where you didn't have time to do anything, including eating a healthy breakfast? You stormed into work one minute before start time and didn't recognize your hunger signals until you reached your desk and started working. After working for a few minutes, you listen to your hunger signals and take a quick stroll into the office kitchen where you find donuts and a cup of coffee. You grab a donut, cup of coffee and indulge in both. All of a sudden, you get this burst of energy and feel like you can attack all of your work in no time.

Before long, you feel like taking a nap and your desk seems like a good place to get some shut eye.

Can you guess what happened?

You have just experienced a sugar crash. Bob, tell her what she has won! Behind door number one, there is a big headache followed by the desire to take a nap and eat more sugar or caffeine to get more energy. Behind door number two is a case of Type 2 diabetes from the continual blood sugar spikes. Finally, behind door number three are 15-20 extra pounds that you will eventually see in the mirror and on the scale. Eating excessive amounts of simple sugars are detrimental to your health and waistline.

Therefore, it is essential to monitor the amount and types of carbohydrates you consume.

You can limit the amount of simple carbohydrates in your diet by ensuring you always have healthy snacks and meals prepared for the workday. Having healthy snacks like fresh fruit, nuts, veggies and lean protein will assist you in making better food choices within your work day.

Rank Your Carbohydrates

Now that you have learned the basic essentials about carbohydrates, let's learn one way to ensure you are eating the right types of carbohydrates without the fear of gaining weight. This can be accomplished by learning how to use the glycemic index.

What is the Glycemic Index?

The "Glycemic Index" is a numerical ranking system which assigns a numeric value to foods based on their immediate rise or effect on blood sugar levels. Foods with a high ranking of 70 and above enter into the blood streams quickly, whereas foods with a ranking of 55 and lower enter into the blood stream at a lower and steady rate. Foods with a high ranking (70 or above) should be eaten sparingly and the majority of your carbohydrates should be chosen from the low ranking category in order to maintain healthy blood sugar levels, weight and to lessen your chance of getting Type 2 diabetes.

In order to use the glycemic index to make healthier food choices, familiarize yourself with the numbers of the foods you currently enjoy eating. If you discover that the majority of your foods come from the higher ranked category, start to discover new foods that appeal to your liking from the lower ranked carbohydrate list. Getting used to new tastes may be a challenge, but in the long run will be beneficial to your health.

Below you will discover a glycemic index for over 100 foods.*

Food	Glycemic Index (glucose = 100)	Serving Size (grams)	Glycemic Load per Serving
BAKERY PRODUCTS AND BREADS			
Banana cake, made with sugar	47	60	14
Banana cake, made without sugar	55	60	12
Sponge cake, plain	46	63	17
Vanilla cake made from packet mix with vanilla frosting (Betty Crocker)	42	111	24
Apple, made with sugar	44	60	13
Apple, made without sugar	48	60	9
Waffles, Aunt Jemima (Quaker Oats)	76	35	10
Bagel, white, frozen	72	70	25
Baguette, white, plain	95	30	15

Food	Glycemic Index (glucose = 100)	Serving Size (grams)	Glycemic Load per Serving
Coarse barley bread, 75-80% kernels, average	34	30	7
Hamburger bun	61	30	9
Kaiser roll	73	30	12
Pumpernickel bread	56	30	7
50% cracked wheat kernel bread	58	30	12
White wheat flour bread	71	30	10
Wonder™ bread, average	73	30	10
Whole wheat bread, average	71	30	9
100% Whole Grain™ bread (Natural Ovens)	51	30	7
Pita bread, white	68	30	10
Corn tortilla	52	50	12
Wheat tortilla	30	50	8
BEVERAGES			
Coca Cola®, average	63	250 mL	16
Fanta®, orange soft drink	68	250 mL	23
Lucozade®, original (sparkling glucose drink)	95±10	250 mL	40
Apple juice, unsweetened, average	44	250 mL	30
Cranberry juice cocktail (Ocean Spray®)	68	250 mL	24
Gatorade	78	250 mL	12
Orange juice, unsweetened	50	250 mL	12
Tomato juice, canned	38	250 mL	4
BREAKFAST CEREALS AND RELATED PRODUCTS			
All-Bran™, average	55	30	12
Coco Pops™, average	77	30	20
Cornflakes™, average	93	30	23
Cream of Wheat™ (Nabisco)	66	250	17
Cream of Wheat™, Instant (Nabisco)	74	250	22
Grapenuts™, average	75	30	16
Muesli, average	66	30	16

Food	Glycemic Index (glucose = 100)	Serving Size (grams)	Glycemic Load per Serving
Oatmeal, average	55	250	13
Instant oatmeal, average	83	250	30
Puffed wheat, average	80	30	17
Raisin Bran™ (Kellogg's)	61	30	12
Special K™ (Kellogg's)	69	30	14
GRAINS			
Pearled barley, average	28	150	12
Sweet corn on the cob, average	60	150	20
Couscous, average	65	150	9
Quinoa	53	150	13
White rice, average	89	150	43
Quick cooking white basmati	67	150	28
Brown rice, average	50	150	16
Converted, white rice (Uncle Ben's®)	38	150	14
Whole wheat kernels, average	30	50	11
Bulgur, average	48	150	12
COOKIES AND CRACKERS			
Graham crackers	74	25	14
Vanilla wafers	77	25	14
Shortbread	64	25	10
Rice cakes, average	82	25	17
Rye crisps, average	64	25	11
Soda crackers	74	25	12
DAIRY PRODUCTS AND ALTERNATIVES			
Ice cream, regular	57	50	6
Ice cream, premium	38	50	3
Milk, full fat	41	250mL	5
Milk, skim	32	250 mL	4
Reduced-fat yogurt with fruit, average	33	200	11
FRUITS			
Apple, average	39	120	6
Banana, ripe	62	120	16

Food	Glycemic Index (glucose = 100)	Serving Size (grams)	Glycemic Load per Serving
Dates, dried	42	60	18
Grapefruit	25	120	3
Grapes, average	59	120	11
Orange, average	40	120	4
Peach, average	42	120	5
Peach, canned in light syrup	40	120	5
Pear, average	38	120	4
Pear, canned in pear juice	43	120	5
Prunes, pitted	29	60	10
Raisins	64	60	28
Watermelon	72	120	4
BEANS AND NUTS			
Baked beans, average	40	150	6
Blackeye peas, average	33	150	10
Black beans	30	150	7
Chickpeas, average	10	150	3
Chickpeas, canned in brine	38	150	9
Navy beans, average	31	150	9
Kidney beans, average	29	150	7
Lentils, average	29	150	5
Soy beans, average	15	150	1
Cashews, salted	27	50	3
Peanuts, average	7	50	0
PASTA and NOODLES			
Fettuccini, average	32	180	15
Macaroni, average	47	180	23
Macaroni and Cheese (Kraft)	64	180	32
Spaghetti, white, boiled, average	46	180	22
Spaghetti, white, boiled 20 min, average	58	180	26
Spaghetti, whole meal, boiled, average	42	180	17

Food	Glycemic Index (glucose = 100)	Serving Size (grams)	Glycemic Load per Serving
SNACK FOODS			
Corn chips, plain, salted, average	42	50	11
Fruit Roll-Ups®	99	30	24
M & M's®, peanut	33	30	6
Microwave popcorn, plain, average	55	20	6
Potato chips, average	51	50	12
Pretzels, oven-baked	83	30	16
Snickers Bar®	51	60	18
VEGETABLES			
Green peas, average	51	80	4
Carrots, average	35	80	2
Parsnips	52	80	4
Baked russet potato, average	111	150	33
Boiled white potato, average	82	150	21
Instant mashed potato, average	87	150	17
Sweet potato, average	70	150	22
Yam, average	54	150	20
MISCELLANEOUS			
Hummus (chickpea salad dip)	6	30	0
Chicken nuggets, frozen, reheated in microwave oven 5 min	46	100	7
Pizza, plain baked dough, served with parmesan cheese and tomato sauce	80	100	22
Pizza, Super Supreme (Pizza Hut)	36	100	9
Honey, average	61	25	12

* "International tables of glycemic index and glycemic load values: 2008" by Fiona S. Atkinson, Kaye Foster-Powell, and Jennie C. Brand-Miller in the December 2008 issue of Diabetes Care, Vol. 31, number 12, pages 2281-2283.

Below are answers to some of the most frequently asked questions regarding carbohydrates.

FAQs Regarding Carbohydrates

Q.

WHAT WILL HAPPEN IF I GO TOO LONG WITHOUT CARBOHYDRATES?

A.

Going too long without a sufficient amount of carbohydrates will cause the body to find other sources of energy to function. This energy may come from protein (muscles) or fat stores. Going long periods of time without a sufficient amount of carbohydrates can cause fatigue and dizziness. The brain and central nervous system need carbohydrates (glucose) in order to function properly, therefore consume carbohydrates in moderation and in the form of complex carbohydrates (whole grains, beans, brown rice and legumes).

Q.

SHOULD I CONSUME CARBOHYDRATES BEFORE I WORK OUT?

A.

Yes. Carbohydrates are the body's main source of energy and the amount you consume before a workout is based on your fitness goal. If your goal is to build lean muscle, you'll need to consume at least 45-50 grams of carbohydrates along with 10-15 grams of protein. If your goal is weight loss, consume at least 25 grams of carbohydrates and 15 grams of protein.

If you're going to consume your carbohydrates in a liquid form, consume it at least 45 minutes prior to your workout. If your source is whole food, allow 90 minutes to 2 hours for food to digest before training. If you exercise for more than an hour, you may need to refuel with a sports energy drink such as Gatorade™ or Powerade™ in order to maintain energy levels. On non-work out days, carbohydrate consumption should be lower. On these days, the body doesn't require as much energy to fuel your body.

Q.

WILL CARBOHYDRATES MAKE ME FAT?

A.

No, not if consumed in moderation and in the form of complex carbohydrates, along with regular physical activity and resistance training. People don't become overweight by just consuming carbohydrates. Weight gain is a combined result of consuming too many calories and limited physical activity.

Q.

IS IT ALRIGHT TO CONSUME SUGAR-FREE PRODUCTS?

A.

Many sugar-free products contain high amounts of synthetic or artificial flavoring and studies have shown some products may cause diarrhea and gastric problems such as bloating and gas. Instead of consuming artificial sweeteners, opt for natural sweeteners that have zero calories. Stevia™ and Truvia™ are a few.

Q.

IF I DON'T WANT TO USE REFINED SUGAR, WHAT IS A GOOD ALTERNATIVE TO SWEETEN FOOD?

A.

There are many natural products on the market such as agave nectar, Stevia™ and Truvia™ that add flavoring and don't cause high sugar spikes. Most of these products are at your local grocery or health food store. You may use these products to bake or sweeten your favorite drinks.

Q.

WHAT IS THE PERCENTAGE OF CARBOHYDRATES SHOULD I CONSUME DAILY?

A.

The amount of carbohydrates you consume on a daily basis is based on your daily physical activity, fitness goals and current weight. If you are an athlete, your intake of carbohydrates may be between 50-60% or higher based on the intensity and duration of your activity. For less active individuals, at least 40 % percent of your diet should come from complex carbohydrate sources.

Q.

HOW DO I CALCULATE THE GRAMS OF CARBOHYDRATES I NEED TO CONSUME ON A DAILY BASIS?

A.

The first step in calculating your required grams is to determine your fitness goals. Do you want to lose weight or do you want to focus more on athletic events and gaining lean muscle? If you want to lose weight, take 40 % of your daily calories to determine carbohydrates in grams. If you want to build lean muscle tissue or you're an athlete, take at least 55 % of your daily calories.

Example: You want to lose weight and you consume 1,600 calories a day

1. Take 1,600 X .40 = 640

2. Take 640/4 (4 = the amount of calories in 1 gram of carbohydrates) = 160

3. Your total daily consumption of carbohydrates equals 160 grams

Example: You want to gain lean muscle or you're athletic and you consume 2,200 calories a day

1. Take 2,200 x. 55 = 1211.

2. Take 1,221 / 4 (4 = the amount of calories in 1 gram of carbohydrates) = 302.5

3. Your total daily consumption of carbohydrates equals 302.5 grams

Chapter

Your body isn't a garbage can, therefore you shouldn't put trash in it!

11

You Are What You Eat

You Are What You Eat!

How many times have you heard this saying?

I would guess too many times to remember. However, my question to you is - have you ever thought about the true meaning of this statement? If you haven't, now is the time to do so.

Now that you are equipped with more information about nutrients, it's time to start thinking about moving forward and making better food choices for you and your family.

As we learned in earlier chapters, eating meals high in saturated fat, sugar and calories can cause health problems and result in weight gain. Therefore, in order to avoid these issues and to get into the best shape of your life, it is important to consider what you are placing into your body.

By no means am I saying you cannot enjoy a hamburger or pizza every now and then. What I am saying is - instead of ordering a pizza or hamburgers why not make your own? Making your own food gives you the ability to control the ingredients and calories. Instead of fatty high calorie meats, you can use lean meats, fat-free cheese and plenty of veggies without the added sodium and preservatives.

If you choose to have a hamburger, why not choose lean meats that are 93% lean (beef, turkey). The leaner the meat, the less fat it will contain and the healthier it will be. In order to add flavoring, you can add olive oil, sea salt, herbs and spices instead of using table salt and other ingredients high in sodium. This method can be applied to all of your favorite foods. Love fried chicken? Why not oven fry it instead of deep frying it in unhealthy oils.

I understand that change is a process, but making small changes such as these

on a weekly basis will add up to better health. Take one week at a time to add a new healthy habit and before you know it, healthy living will become second nature.

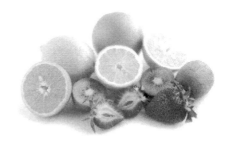

Top 5 Healthy Eating Guidelines

Prepare food in advance: Preparing food in advance will provide you with healthy food available at all times (work and home). This will help minimize the impulse to stop for fast food or other unhealthy snacks when you're hungry. Portion off healthy snacks and carry with you at all times.

Eat every 2-3 hours: Eating small meals more frequently throughout the day will keep your blood sugar levels even and ward off hunger. Eating more frequently will in addition help you avoid consuming to many calories at one meal.

Drink water throughout the day: Over 65 percent of your body is water. Consuming water throughout the day will keep you full and help transport toxins and waste from your body and help curb hunger.

Snack in between meals: Snacking in between meals will keep the hunger monster away and prevent you from consuming large meals at one sitting.

Limit eating out: Eating out can be expensive and add inches to your waistline and hips. Therefore if you decide to eat out, eat out only 1 time per week and go to places that have healthier options on their menu. Request to have salad dressings on the side and don't be afraid to ask for a to go box for left overs.

Don't Believe the Hype

Learning how to eat healthy can be a mystery based on the fact that there are so many products on the grocery market shelves whose packages boast their products to be healthy, when in actuality they aren't as healthy as their packaging would like to boast.

Marketing companies often create extraordinary visuals to grab consumer's eyes and doing so leaves a great opportunity to entice consumers with beautiful packaging and fancy words without really telling what's completely in the food product. If you're like many shoppers, more than likely you have fallen for this marketing hype at least once in your life.

Let me show you how this all works. Take a moment and walk with me down grocery lane.

One day you find yourself wandering down the grocery aisle and you pass by a bottle of fruit juice. Based on its enticing words like 100% Daily Serving of Vitamin C and that big word, ANTIOXIDANT, you put it in your cart without reading the nutrition or ingredient label. The pretty picture of fresh fruit splashed across the bottle gave you a sense of fruit heaven and if you had a glass available, you would have poured yourself a serving or two.

You finally make it home and want a glass of your fruit juice, but before pouring a glass you turn the bottle over to read the nutrition label and you find out that your fruit juice really isn't all fruit juice. At the top of the bottle, you see a sign that says it contains 10% fruit juice. Oh no! You mean this beautiful bottle really doesn't contain all the fruit it

claimed by its array of pretty fruit on the front of the bottle?

You got it, and you have just bought into the marketing hype. Don't feel bad, you are not alone. Many people buy food items based on what they see on the front of the package instead of turning over the products and reading the nutrition and ingredient labels.

No worries, long gone are the days when you pick up a food product and think it's healthy based on the appearance of the package. It's time to learn how to read nutrition and ingredient labels and make better food choices.

Read All Labels

What are nutrition facts and ingredient labels?

Nutrition facts and ingredient labels are labels located on food products that list nutrients by their daily percentages and ingredients by their weight. Making the decision not to read these labels and strictly depend on advertisement alone can be misleading. Learning how to read these labels will empower you to know what you are really consuming. Let's learn how to read ingredient and nutrition labels.

Explore the Labels

As you learn to eat healthier, a new guideline for grocery shopping involves not placing any food items into your cart without first reading the nutrition facts and ingredient list label. If it's an unpackaged product (such as fresh fruit or vegetables), it's OK to place these items into your cart. Sticking to this guideline will keep you be more aware of the food choices you are making and help you get accustomed to reading food labels. Yes, this may be more time-consuming, but your health is worth it.

Where do you begin?

First, locate the nutrition facts label on the product. The majority of products list this information either on the back or side of the food item. The nutrition facts label informs you of the amount of a certain nutrient you will consume from a particular product (protein, saturated fat, sodium). Once you have located this label, proceed to follow these steps.

Locate the serving size and the number of servings in the package. Serving sizes are standard in order to compare similar foods. They are listed in units, such as cups or pieces, followed by the metric unit, e.g.. the number of grams. Pay close attention to serving sizes. The more servings in the package equals more calories consumed.

Locate the amount of calories per serving. If you find a package that says 250 calories, but you fail to see that the entire package has two servings and eat the entire package, you are getting 250 more calories for a total of 500 calories.

Look at calories and percentages for fat, carbohydrates, protein, sodium and cholesterol. The nutrition facts label will list these items in grams per serving. Follow your guidelines when it comes to fat. The majority of your calories should come from unsaturated fat. Limit products that are high in saturated and

trans fats. In addition to these bad sources of fat, stay away from foods that are high in sodium. Foods with more than 20 percent of your daily value of sodium should be avoided.

Look at the percentages of vitamins and minerals. Underneath the list of macro-nutrients you will find a list of vitamins and minerals with their percentages. These percentages are based on the amounts food in the food item.

Once you have read the nutrition facts label, you will look for the ingredients list label. Legally, every food product is required to list all ingredients that were used to make the particular product. Food products normally list ingredients by weight, therefore by reading the ingredient list you are more aware of what is truly in a product.

If you were reading an ingredient list, you would focus on the first five ingredients. Since ingredients are listed by weight, the products that are listed first in the list are the bulk of the product. If the first ingredient is sugar, most of that product is sugar. Even though the nutrition label may state that there are only 7 grams of sugar in this product, pay attention to the ingredient list. I stress again, if sugar is the first ingredient on the list, the majority of the product is sugar.

When reading ingredient lists, a rule of thumb to remember is if you can't pronounce the word, more than likely it is a chemical or preservative and you don't want that in your body.

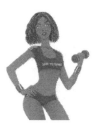

FIT JEWEL

Try to find products that have shorter ingredient lists and are as natural as possible.

Try to find products that have shorter ingredient lists and are as natural as possible. By doing this, you lessen the chance of putting excessive amounts of unhealthy products in your body.

An example of a food ingredient list may look like this:

Ingredients: sugar, water, salt, high fructose corn syrup, partially hydrogenated vegetable oil

Information that must be listed on all food product packaging includes:

Product information

A list of ingredients

Name of food

Net weight

Nutritional content

The name and address of the manufacturer

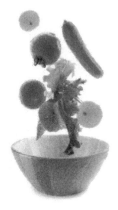

Nutritional Overload

You may feel overwhelmed with all of this information, but keep in mind getting healthy is a process with many destinations. Take your time and learn at your own pace. Getting healthy isn't a sprint.

Below you will find answers to three of the most frequently asked questions regarding calories.

FAQs Regarding Calories

Q.

HOW MANY CALORIES SHOULD I EAT ON A DAILY BASIS?

A.

The amount of calories you need to consume is based on factors such as gender, age, physical activity, current weight and fitness goals. The first factor is gender. When it comes to caloric needs, men require a higher amount of calories than women. Women have less body mass, therefore require fewer calories.

The next factor is age. Generally, as we age, we tend to decrease our physical activity, which means our bodies require fewer calories.

As for current weight, if you desire to gain weight, you will consume more calories than a person trying to lose weight will. If you want to lose weight, consume less calories and increase your physical activity to burn more calories than you consume. By doing this, you will create a caloric deficit and lose weight.

The last and most important factor is activity level. If you are an inactive person, your caloric intake will be different from someone who works out five days per week. An active person will consume a higher amount of calories that are needed for energy. Therefore, in order to determine your daily caloric requirement it is essential to determine your goals, current weight and activity level.

Once you have this data, follow the chart below to get a general idea of how many calories you need to consume on a daily basis. The numbers below are just a generalization. Adapt your caloric consumption based on your individual needs.

Recommended Calorie (Energy) Intake for Females			
Age	Light Activity	Moderate Activity	Heavy Activity
11-18	2,000	2,100	2,600
19-24	2,000	2,300	2,800
25-50	2,200	2,300	2,800
51+	1,900		

Classification of Activity Levels

Very Light: Typing, sewing, cross word puzzles, video games

Light: Gardening, garage work, golf, table tennis

Moderately Active: Walking, weeding, hoeing, bike riding, hiking

Heavy: Cycling, heavy resistance training, power lifting, sprinting

Q.

WHEN SHOULD I EAT MY FIRST MEAL TO CONSUME ALL OF MY CALORIES?

A.

Since you were a child, you probably have heard that breakfast is the most important meal of the day. I will reiterate what you have heard. Breakfast is the most important meal of the day. At night, we average 7-8 hours of sleep and by the time we eat our last meal and awake, our bodies have gone without food for approximately 10-11 hours.

In the morning we are in a catabolic (breaking down) state and need to re-fuel our bodies. During the morning, our bodies are seeking healthy nutrients to prepare us for the day. If you are one of those people who say, "I don't have time for breakfast" my response to that is, you can't afford not to make time for breakfast. Studies have shown people who eat breakfast are more likely to lose weight and keep it off versus those who skip breakfast. As a guideline, eat within 1 hour of waking up.

Q.

SHOULD I STOP EATING AFTER 6 P.M.?

A.

No. If you are on a daily nutrition plan that consists of consuming 2,000 calories a day and by 6 pm you have only consumed 1,400 calories, your body my still require more calories. Skipping out on 600 calories can leave you hungry and cause you to eat more calories at your next meal. Therefore when you recognize hunger, feed your body even if it is after 6:00 pm. If you do so, your meals should consist of a source of lean protein and at least 3 servings of vegetables. Late in the evenings your body doesn't need a large amount of carbohydrates. You can consume your carbohydrates by eating vegetables.

Friend vs. Foe

You have learned a lot of information in the previous chapters, so let's take a quick moment to exhale. Whew. Alright, is your mind clear now? If it is, let's continue to move forward.

We need to move forward and talk about something that keeps many women from reaching their fitness and weight loss goals. What we need to address is your relationship with food.

Women often find themselves on a vicious cycle of a love-hate relationship with food. Some women are dieters who go through a constant battle of weight gain and weight loss, only to find themselves lost in a sea of disappointment and pounds heavier. At the other end of the spectrum, there are women who want to enjoy food but are too consumed with the fear of gaining weight and as a result, they either purge (bulimia) or deny themselves food (anorexia).

Do you fit into either one of these categories?

If you do, it is important to realize that you have the power to start a healthy relationship with food. Eating should be an enjoyable process, but in order for this to happen, it is essential that you get to the root cause of why you and food have the relationship that you have. Maybe you're an emotional eater and learned these eating habits during your childhood. If you're an emotional eater, you will be challenged with learning new ways to cope with your emotions. It is

important that we use food to fuel our bodies and not to suppress or address our emotions. It may be scary to address the issues that you have suppressed, but doing so will free you from this pattern of behavior.

Whatever your situation, you have to start peeling back the layers in order to find answers to your relationship with food.

Do you find yourself eating if you are happy, sad, bored, alone or excited?

Are you eating to fill a void? If you are, have you ever asked yourself why?

Take Control of Your Eating

If you are struggling with food, find someone you can confide in and let them be your support system, this support system may include a licensed psychologist who specializes in eating disorders. Be open with whomever you share your fears and concerns with; doing so will shed light onto a sometimes dark issue.

After being honest with yourself and sharing this information with someone you trust, you may discover the root cause(s) of why you feel the way you do about food.

In the process of this discovery, keep a food journal in order to track how much, when, and what times of the day you are eating. Write down any emotions felt during the times you are eating. At the end of the week, review your journal and look for certain foods attached to certain moods and behaviors. The unveiling of this information can be life-altering.

I can't guarantee this process will be easy, but with consistent effort, patience and discipline, you can change old behaviors and accomplish your weight loss and fitness goals.

Daily Caloric Tracking Sheet

Tracking your meals and snacks will help to keep you conscience of your daily caloric consumption. Monitor your moods before and after your meals, this may help identify food triggers.

Sun: [ ] Mon: [ ] Tues: [ ] Wed: [ ] Thurs: [ ] Fri: [ ] Sat: [ ]

Weight: [ ]   Date: [ ]

Weekly Eating Goal(s)

Place	Time of Day	Food/ Beverage	Calories	Mood Before	Mood After

Daily Calorie Intake:

What were you feeling today? (Happy, sad, excited, bored, lonely, angry, depressed, jealous, determined, persistent etc.)

Water consumption:

Daily Overview (triggers you discovered, patterns in eating, types of foods most craved, etc.):

Do You Have A Healthy Relationship With Food?

Take time to answer each question honestly. The answers to these questions are for your eyes only and may reveal important information to you regarding your eating habits and patterns.

Date:

1. Do you skip breakfast on a regular basis?

2. Do you eat even when you are not hungry?

3. Do you eat when you are happy, sad, bored, alone or excited?

4. Do you listen to your body's hunger signals or do you ignore them?

5. Do you feel bad about eating in front of others?

6. Do you enjoy fresh fruits, whole grains and veggies regularly?

7. Are you frequently on a diet?

8. Do you consume too many empty calories (alcohol), soda or energy drinks?

9. Do you eat every 2-3 hours?

10. Do you deny yourself food when you are hungry?

11. Do you eat while working?

12. Do you enjoy taking your time and eating slowly?

13. Do you need to be more consistent with meal timing?

14. Do you need to eat more?

15. Do you need to cut back on calories?

16. Are you an emotional eater?

Keep your answers to yourself or find a support system to help you get on track with healthy and mindful eating. Find other health conscience people to encourage and give you an example to model.

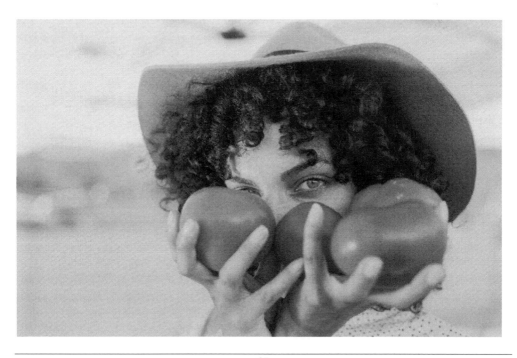

Tools of Success

Defining your curves and becoming healthy is a lifelong process. Therefore, on your way to achieving your fitness goals, pack the following tips in your purse, gym bag or lunch box:

Never skip breakfast: Skipping breakfast will cause you to become hungry throughout the day and consume extra calories. Start your day off right by having a healthy breakfast.

Always keep healthy snacks available: Keeping healthy snacks available will keep you from eating office junk food or visiting a snack machine whenever you are hungry. Use snack bags to portion off snacks like fresh cut fruit, vegetables and nuts.

Increase your fiber intake. Fiber keeps you full and helps regulate healthy bowel movements. Fiber is the indigestible part of food that helps remove waste from the digestive track.

Do not eat when bored or stressed: Emotional eating can add pounds to your frame. If you are going through a tough time, take a minute before you eat and ask yourself are you hungry or are you eating to sooth a particular emotion. If you're not hungry, go for a brisk walk or find a good book to read.

Eat small, frequent meals throughout the day every 2-3 hours: Eating frequently throughout the day will prevent hunger and drops in your blood sugar levels.

Limit your amount of alcohol. Alcohol is full of empty calories and can increase caloric intake. Drink sparingly and in moderation.

Eat complete meals: Eating a complete meal involves including a source of protein, fat and a complex carbohydrate (whole grains). Eating complete meals will keep you full longer and provide your body essential nutrients.

If you have a family, make a group decision to make healthier food choices: A rule of thumb: if you shouldn't eat unhealthy food, neither should your family. Making a family decision will make the transition easier and beneficial to the entire family.

Be aware of food portions: Eating large portions of food can cause weight gain. Therefore, purchase a weight scale and weigh your food until you train your eye to determine true size proportions. Eating with smaller plates can help give you a visual aid.

If you fall off the health wagon, start over fresh the next day: If you get off track with your healthy eating, don't throw in the towel. Guilt will not help get you back on track. Address your barriers and move forward.

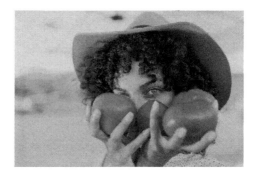

Limit your intake of processed and canned foods: Processed and canned foods contain high amounts of sodium and chemicals which, if consumed in large amounts, can lead to water retention (edema) and high blood pressure (hypertension). Limit these products and purchase fresh or frozen.

When grocery shopping, shop the perimeter of the store: By shopping on the perimeter of the grocery store you will find fresh fruits, vegetables and other healthy products. Shopping in the middle aisles is where the majority of processed and canned foods are located.

Always read nutrition labels: Read all nutrition facts and ingredient list labels. Don't be fooled by pretty packaging and creative wording.

Consider food as fuel for the body. Look at food as fuel and this will help you make better food choices: Without proper fuel (food) the body doesn't function the way it was designed and you gain excessive amounts of weight.

Prepare meals in advance: Preparing meals in advance will help you avoid making impulsive food decisions. Try to avoid leaving your house without healthy meals or snacks on a daily basis.

Take time and chew your food slowly: Chewing your food slowly will allow you to enjoy the taste of your food and give you a sense of fullness. Don't eat while working, step away from your work and enjoy your food.

Avoid foods high in saturated and trans fat: Consuming foods high in saturated and trans fat can lead to high cholesterol, heart disease, obesity and many other health risks. Eat these foods sparingly.

Use condiments sparingly: Ketchup and creamy salad dressings can be high in sugar and calories and offer little-to-no nutritional value. Get creative and make your own seasonings by using herbs, olive oil and sea salt.

Start each meal with small amounts of food on your plate: Start off by eating small amounts of food. Eat what is on your plate and then take a few minutes to decide if you are still hungry.

If the answer is yes, then go back for another small portion of food.

Choose lean sources of protein: Lean sources of meat have less fat and are healthier. Therefore, choose sources at least 93 % lean.

Choose complex carbohydrates: Choosing complex carbohydrates such as whole grains, brown rice, quinoa, and steel cuts oats over simple sugars (cakes, donuts, crackers) can help maintain your blood sugar levels and ward off the hunger monster.

Buy frozen or fresh fruits and vegetables: Buying foods that are fresh or frozen or in their most natural state are healthier than boxed or processed foods. Eat boxed and processed food sparingly.

Reduce sodium intake: Consuming high amounts of sodium can cause health issues such as hypertension. Therefore, instead of using salt, season food with spices and herbs. If you choose to use salt, sea salt is a healthier alternative.

Drink sufficient amounts of water: More than 60 percent of the body is made of water. Water is used for weight loss, to carry nutrients to cells, cushion joints and to regulate body temperature and blood pressure. Therefore, consume at least 2.2 liters (9 cups per day). If you exercise, drink water before, during and after your work outs. Being dehydrated (lack of water intake) can cause fatigue and affect your optimal exercise performance.

Chapter

Your body is a machine and needs to be fueled properly to function right.

12

Feed the Machine

It's Not a Diet, It's a Lifestyle

This chapter provides you with easy to prepare, palate pleasing recipes for breakfast, lunch, dinner and snacks. The nutritional content and calories counts for each meal are listed on each recipe card. In order to give you a generalized idea of what to eat within a day, a sample meal plan for 1,600, 1,800 and 2,000 calorie meal plans is provided. Do not forget to eat every 2-3 hours and track your meals to determine your daily caloric intake.

Eat, enjoy and thrive!

Breakfast

Breakfast is the most important meal of the day and shouldn't be skipped. Eating a balanced amount of calories during this time of the day will fuel your body for the remainder of the day and leave you less hungry. Studies have shown people who eat breakfast on a consistent basis are more likely to manage their weight. The meals below provide you with variety and flavor.

Below are your options for breakfast.

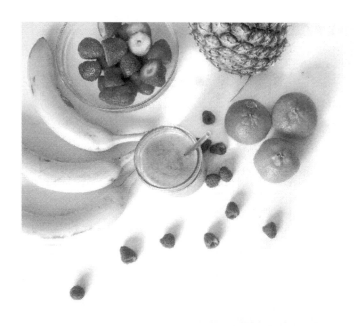

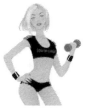

FIT JEWEL

Eating a healthy breakfast will fuel the beginning of your day and prevent you from consuming excess calories throughout the day

CINNAMON NUT OATMEAL

Ingredients:
½ cup Steel Cut Oatmeal
½ oz Slivered Almonds
Cinnamon (use to your liking. Cinnamon has many health benefits minus the calories)
Agave Nectar (few drops)

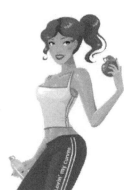

Preparation:
1. Boil 1 cup of water and place oats into water.
2. Cook for 3-5 minutes.
3. In a bowl, add slivered almonds, a few drops of Agave Nectar and cinnamon and mix together.
4. Once oatmeal is cooked, place mix on top.

Total calories 232, protein 8 g, carbohydrates 29.8 g, fat 1.5 g

To add more protein, add two egg whites to meal for an additional 34 calories and 7 g of protein.

PUMPKIN SPICE FRENCH TOAST

Ingredients:
1 or 2 pieces of Ezekiel Bread
1 whole egg
2 egg whites
Pumpkin Spice
Nutmeg
Few drops of Agave Nectar
Pam non stick spray

Preparation:
1. Crack one whole egg and two egg whites into a bowl, add cinnamon and nutmeg, then mix.
2. Place bread into egg mix. Allow each side to absorb mix for about 1 minute.
3. Use a medium sized skillet, cover bottom of pan with Pam. Add bread to skillet.
4. Cook on each side until brown. Once done, add a few drops of Agave Nectar on each side in the pan. Allow bread to caramelize before taking out of skillet.

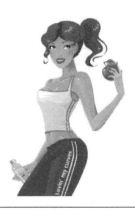

Total calories 220, protein 12 g, carbohydrates 30, fat 5 g

To add more protein to this meal, add 3 slices of low-sodium turkey bacon 35 calories per slice equals 105 kcal.

BREAKFAST BURRITOS

Ingredients:

2 whole eggs
1 egg white
½ bell pepper
½ tomato
½ onion

1 whole wheat tortilla
Pam non stick spray
1 slice non- fat cheese
2 Tbsp. salsa
Salt and pepper

Preparation:
1. Chop bell pepper, tomato, onion, and place in a bowl.
2. Crack whole eggs and egg white into bowl with veggies, add salt and pepper, mix.
3. In a medium size skillet, cover bottom of skillet with Pam non-stick spray and add egg mix.
4. Scramble until eggs are to your liking.
5. Take tortilla and add fat-free cheese, place egg mix on top then wrap. Place salsa on top (optional).

Total Calories 300, protein 14 g, carbohydrates 19 g, fat 12g

Add 2 slices of low sodium bacon that adds another 70 calories. You may also add ½ glass of all-natural 100 percent fruit juice.

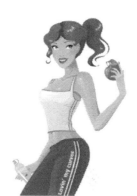

BREAKFAST BAGEL

Ingredients:

1 whole wheat bagel
2 egg whites
3 tomato slices
1/2 slice fat-free cheese
½ Tbsp. light mayonnaise
Pam non stick spray

Preparation:
1. Spray skillet with Pam non-stick spray. Crack egg and cook until done
2. Slice tomato into 1-inch slices.
3. Cut bagel in half and place in toaster until browned. Remove bagel from toaster and spread light mayonnaise onto both pieces of bread. Add cheese and tomatoes on one-half.
4. Once egg is done add egg to bagel.

Total Calories 340, protein 15g, carbohydrates 35 g, fat 6.5 g

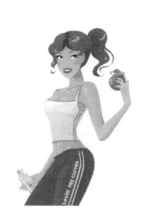

Lunch or Dinner Choices

The following meals can be eaten for either lunch or dinner - you make the choice. Just like breakfast, don't skip lunch.

Lunch
Lunch is a time to refuel your body for the remainder of the work day, which will help stave off the hunger monster and your cravings for unhealthy snacks.

If you are like most people who enjoy eating out during the workday, plan ahead and make wise food choices. Call the restaurant ahead of time in order to determine if they offer a healthy options menu. By doing this, you can plan what you are going to eat before your arrival to the restaurant. If portion sizes at the restaurant are large, don't be afraid to ask for a to-go-box and split half of your meal for later.

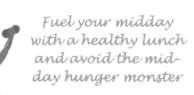

FIT JEWEL

*Fuel your midday
with a healthy lunch
and avoid the mid-
day hunger monster*

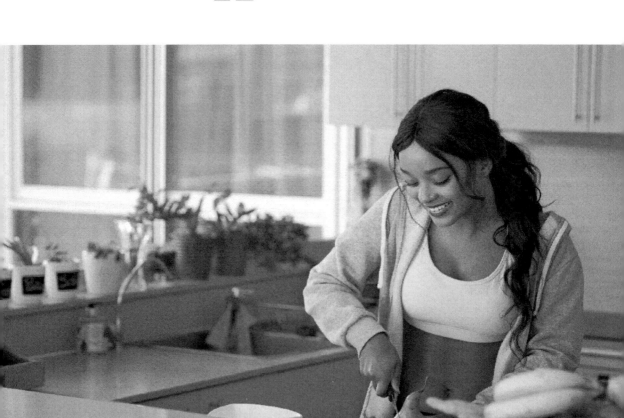

Dinner

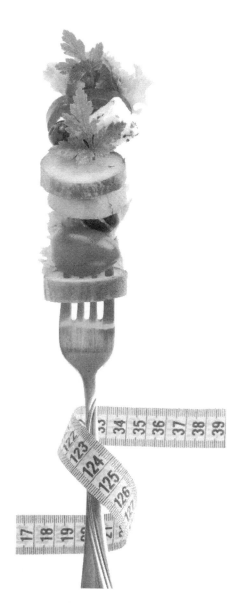

Dinner is the last full meal of the day and shouldn't consist of more than 350 calories. By this time of the day, if you have eaten every 2-3 hours, the hunger monster shouldn't be too hard to handle. If you have missed eating your required calories during the day, be aware of the amount of calories you consume before bedtime. Eating a large meal will pack the pounds on. If you are hungry before bed, have a light snack and drink a glass of caffeine free tea or water to give you a sense of being full. When choosing meals for dinner time, it is recommended to choose meals that are lower in carbohydrates. As the body slows down its activity level towards the latter part of the day, we don't need as many carbohydrates. All calories that are not used as energy are converted and stored as fat. Therefore, be aware of your caloric intake before bed.

Enjoy these flavorful and palate pleasing recipes and don't be afraid to add extra vegetables for more nutrients and fiber.

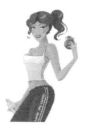

FIT JEWEL

Eat great,
feel great,
look great!

TUNA QUESADILLAS

Ingredients:
1 -5 oz. can tuna (in water)
Whole wheat tortilla
½ cup tomatoes
½ scallions

2 Tbsp. salsa
½ Tbsp. of mayonnaise
1 slice fat-free cheese

Preparation:
1. Drain tuna, mix mayonnaise with tuna.
2. Chop tomatoes and scallions.
3. Spray skillet with non-stick Pam spray. Place one tortilla in skillet then place tuna mix in middle of tortilla.
4. Add cheese on top of tuna mix. Add second tortilla on top. Brown one side then flip to other side. Cut quesadilla into four triangles. Add salsa on top.
5. Add a side salad with fat free dressing and plenty of veggies to complete meal.

Total Calories 345, protein 21g, carbohydrates 32 g, fat 12 g

In order to cut back on calories, only consume half of quesadilla and prepare 2 servings of vegetables which is 1 cup of vegetables of your liking. You may also prepare a salad to add with half serving

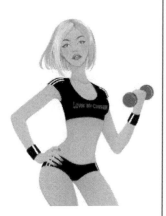

TUNA MELT

Ingredients:
1- 5 oz. can tuna (in water)
½ Tbsp. mayonnaise
2 slices whole wheat bread
2 slices tomatoes

Preparation:
1. Drain tuna, add mayonnaise, mix.
2. Lightly spread olive oil spread on both sides of bread. Place bread in heated skillet. Place tuna mix in middle of bread and place tomatoes on top of mix. Place second piece of bread on top.
3. Cook until brown on both sides. Brown both sides to your liking. Cut in half and serve.

Total calories 406, protein 33g, carbohydrates 40 g, fat 10 g

To cut back on carbohydrates and calories, use thinly sliced bread or a pita pocket.

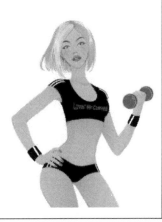

TURKEY BURRITOS

Ingredients:

4 oz. ground turkey	1 slice fat-free cheese
1 whole wheat tortilla	½ Tbsp. olive oil
½ chopped tomato	1 Tbsp. sour cream
½ onion	2 Tbsp. salsa

Preparation:

1. Add ½ Tbsp. of olive oil to a heated skillet. Season turkey meat with selected seasoning, and then add meat to skillet. Once meat begins to cook, add onions. Brown meat until fully cooked.
2. Slightly brush olive oil on front and back of tortilla. Place tortilla in microwave for 20 seconds. Do over cook or tortilla will become too hard.
3. Take tortilla and place fat free cheese in middle, add turkey mix, then wrap.
4. Place chopped tomatoes, fat-free sour cream and salsa on top of wrap.

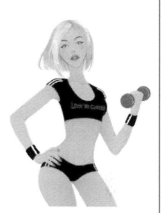

Total calories 440 calories, protein 38g, carbohydrates 35 g, 9.5 g fat

For less calories, cut burrito in half and save remaining half for later.

TURKEY EXTRAVAGANZA

Ingredients:

4 oz. Turkey Sausage	½ red onion
2/3 cup whole wheat Penne pasta	2 Tbsp. fat-free Italian Dressing
½ green pepper	1 Tbsp. olive oil
½ red pepper	

Preparation:

1. Heat water until water comes to boil. Add pasta and cook for 5-7 min. Do not overcook pasta.
2. Cut sausage into 1-inch slices. Chop green peppers, red peppers and onions into 1-inch slices. In a medium size bowl, add all ingredients together.
3. Add one Tbsp. of olive oil to a medium sized pan. Once oil is heated, add sausage, bell peppers and onions to pan. Allow mix to sauté for 7-10 minutes. Do not overcook.
4. Once mix is finished sautéing, add two Tbsp. of fat-free Italian dressing and mix.
5. Drain pasta then add mix on top of pasta.

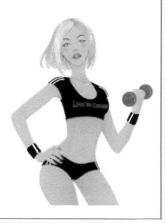

Total calories 450, protein 24 g, carbohydrates 35 g, fat 10 g

SPINACH SUNRISE SALAD

Ingredients:
4 oz. Chicken breast
4 cups baby spinach
½ apple
½ cup mandarin oranges
¼ cup walnuts
1 Tbsp. Raspberry Vinegar Dressing

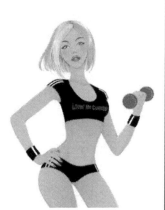

Preparation:
1. Grill or bake chicken and cut chicken into 1-inch slices, or use 4 oz. precooked chicken strips.
2. Chop apples into square pieces.
3. In a bowl mix, walnuts, oranges, apple pieces and salad dressing.
4. Add mix to baby spinach.

Total calories 350, protein 23g, carbohydrates 40 g, fat 3g

SUNDRIED TOMATO WRAP

Ingredients:
1 sun dried tomato wrap
3 slices deli roast beef
3 slices turkey breast
½ Tbsp. Ranch Dressing
3 tomato slices
1 slice fat-free cheese

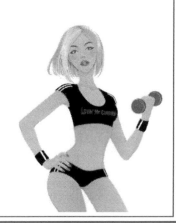

Preparation:
1. Place cheese on the bottom of tortilla. Place roast beef and turkey breast on top of cheese.
2. Place in microwave for 20 seconds to heat.
3. Spread dressing on top of meat then add tomatoes.
4. Wrap and cut in half.

Total calories 325, protein 24 g, carbohydrates 35 g,
fat 11.5 g

Eating healthy is about moderation, not deprivation.

Snacks can be from 100-200 calories. Snacking in between meals will keep your blood sugar levels stable and help you avoid overeating. Get creative and enjoy!

DARK CHOCOLATE STRAWBERRIES

Ingredients:

½ cup trimmed strawberries
½ dark chocolate
4-5 toothpicks

Preparation:

1. Melt dark chocolate.
2. Thoroughly rinse strawberries and cut off stems.
3. Insert toothpicks into strawberries.
4. Dip strawberries into dark chocolate.

Approximately 100-150 calories, depending on chocolate.

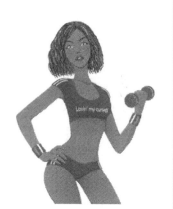

FLAVORED POPCORN

Ingredients:

1 snack bag natural light popcorn
Choice of seasoning (Parmesan, Cinnamon sugar, Cheyenne Pepper, Hot Sauce)

Preparation:

1. Pop popcorn.
2. Sprinkle seasoning onto popcorn, close bag, then shake.

Approximately 100 calories.

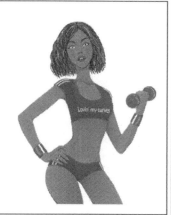

BAGEL AND CREAM CHEESE

Ingredients:

½ whole wheat bagel
2 Tbsp. fat-free cream cheese (flavored)
1 serving low fat spread

Preparation:
1. Cut bagel in half; wrap other half for later use.
2. Lightly spread low-fat spread on bagel, then place bagel into toaster.
3. Toast bagel until lightly brown. Remove from toaster and add cream cheese.

Approximately 115 calories.

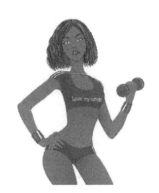

CHOCOLATE RICE CAKE AND PEANUT BUTTER

Ingredients:

2 rice cakes
1 Tbsp. peanut butter

Preparation:

1. Spread ½ tablespoon of peanut butter on each rice cake.
2. Eat and enjoy.

Approximately 175 calories.

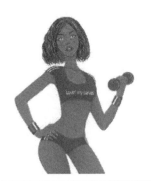

HUMMUS AND WHOLE GRAIN CHIPS

Ingredients:

½ cup whole wheat crackers (lower sodium)
2 Tbsp. hummus (plain or flavored)

Preparation:

1. Spread hummus onto whole grain crackers.
2. Eat and enjoy.

Approximately 150 calories.

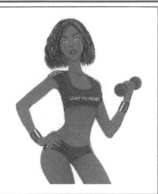

APPLE AND CHEESE STICK

Ingredients:

1 medium sized apple
2% milk string cheese

Preparation:

1.   Thoroughly wash apple. Eat apple with cheese.

Approximately 165 calories.

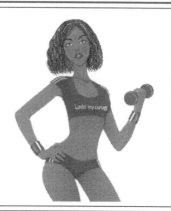

SWEET POTATO FRIES

Ingredients:

1 medium sized potato
Pam non- stick spray
Pinch of salt

Preparation:

1.   Preheat oven to 350 degrees for 5-6 minutes.
2.   Thoroughly wash outside of potato.
3.   Cut potato into fours.
4.   Cut each fourth into 1-inch slices.
5.   Sprinkle pinch of salt on potatoes and mix.
6.   Spray non-stick pan with Pam spray.
7.   Add potatoes to pan.
8.   Cook until brown. Rotate potatoes once or twice to brown each side.

Approximately 120 Calories

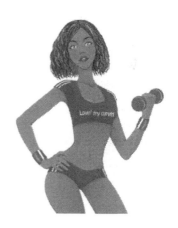

CHOCOLATE STRAWBERRY SOY SHAKE

Ingredients:

1 cup chocolate soy milk
½ fresh strawberries
4-5 ice cubes (optional)

Preparation:

1. Trim and thoroughly clean strawberries.
2. Pour cup of soymilk into blender. Add strawberries and ice.
3. Blend. Pour mix into cup.

Approximately 125 calories.

To get more protein in this snack, add one scoop of chocolate or plain whey protein.

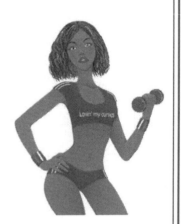

PEANUT BUTTER HONEY WRAP

Ingredients:

½ whole wheat tortilla wrap
½ medium banana
1 Tbsp. peanut butter
Few drops of honey

Preparation:

1. Cut whole tortilla wrap in half, and then cut banana in half.
2. Spread peanut butter onto tortilla and then spread honey on top of peanut butter.
3. Place banana in middle of tortilla then wrap.

Approximately 225 calories

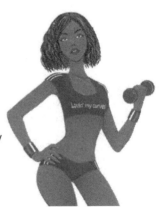

Sample Meal Plans

The following meal plans are samples of **1,600**, **1,800** and **2,000** calories. These meal plans are just an example of how to plan your day based on your daily caloric intake.

As a rule of thumb, consume your first meal within one hour from the time you awake and eat every 2-3 hours thereafter. Eating every 2-3 hours will fuel your body on a consistent basis and relieve hunger and cravings.

Sample Meal Plan for 1,600 Calories

Meal # 1
Breakfast: Breakfast Burrito = 220 calories
½ avocado = 60 calories
4 oz almond milk = 30 calories

Snack # 1
1 small sized apple = 95 calories
1 2% milk string cheese = 70 calories

Meal # 2
Lunch: Sundried Tomato Wrap = 325 calories
1 small garden salad with 1 tbsp fat-free dressing = 45 calories

Snack #2
1/3 cup serving of almonds = 160 calories

Meal # 3
Dinner: Spinach Sunrise Salad = 350 calories
1 glass decaffeinated tea = 2 calories

Snack # 3
Chocolate Strawberry Soy Shake = 125 calories
1 120-calorie pistachio snack = 120 calories

Sample Meal Plan for 1,800 Calories

Meal # 1
Breakfast: Breakfast Bagel = 340 calories
½ avocado = 60 calories
4 oz almond milk = 30 calories

Snack # 1
1 small sized apple = 95 calories
1 2% milk string cheese = 70 calories

Meal # 2
Lunch: Sundried Tomato Wrap = 325 calories
1 small garden salad with 1 tbsp fat-free dressing = 45 calories

Snack #2
1/3 cup serving of almonds = 160 calories
5 celery sticks = 75 calories

Meal # 3
Dinner: Spinach Sunrise Salad = 350 calories
1 glass decaffeinated tea = 2 calories

Snack # 3
Chocolate Strawberry Soy Shake = 125 calories
1 120-calorie pistachio snack = 120 calories

A healthy, well-balanced meal with healthy sources of fat, protein and complex carbohydrates are essential to your weight loss and health.

Meal # 1
Breakfast: Banana Nut Oatmeal =
232 calories
2 egg whites = 35 calories
4 oz almond milk = 30 calories

Snack # 1
1 small sized apple = 95 calories
1 2% milk string cheese = 70 calories

Meal # 2
Lunch: Sundried Tomato Wrap =
325 calories
1 small garden salad with 1 tbsp fat–
free dressing = 45 calories

Snack #2
1/3 cup serving of almonds =
160 calories
5 celery sticks = 75 calories

Meal # 3
Dinner: Spinach Sunrise Salad =
350 calories
1 glass decaffeinated tea = 2 calories

Snack # 3
Chocolate Strawberry Soy Shake =
125 calories
1 120-calorie pistachio snack =
120 calories

Meal #4
½ Turkey Burrito = 220 calories
1 garden side salad = 45 calories

It's a Family Affair

Creating healthy meals for yourself and your family can be challenging - especially in today's fast paced busy world. As a busy mom, sometimes drive-thru my seem more convenient, but do not be fooled by amazing marketing. Fast food isn't healthy for you or your family.

You and your family deserve to eat meals that nourish your body and health. Therefore, let's explore how you and your family can get healthy together.

How can you make the process of healthy eating easier for you and the family?

Have your family assist you in making healthy menus. Creating healthy menus as a family will get your family involved in the healthy eating process and will allow you to spend valuable time together.

Find out what your family likes to eat: Changing unhealthy eating behaviors may be difficult at first, but allow your children to try different healthy foods until they find what they like. Do not force them to eat foods they do not enjoy. There are many healthy choices out there; be patient, they will eventually decide which foods they like.

Allow your kids to help prepare and cook healthy meals with you: I know sometimes you are in a hurry and want to get dinner done, but having your children involved will teach them how to cook and once again, you are spending valuable time with them.

Make a family commitment to live healthier: Making a family commitment to get healthy makes the process more enjoyable when everyone's in it together. Hold each other accountable and support one another. Becoming healthier is a process and it will not happen overnight, but the process is much easier if you have support from the people who love you the most.

Once a month, try one new food item: Don't get stuck in a healthy food rut. Adding a new fruit, grain, veggie or lean meat will provide your palate with new taste and texture. Healthy eating should be fun and enjoyable. Inspire your kids and show them you are also open to new foods. You are their best role model.

Menu Planning Sheet

Copy the following sheet and use it to plan your weekly meals. Having a plan of action for your weekly meals will keep you focused on clean eating. Get creative and try new healthy foods.

Day: _____ **Date:** _____

Breakfast:

Lunch:

Dinner:

Snacks:

Part III

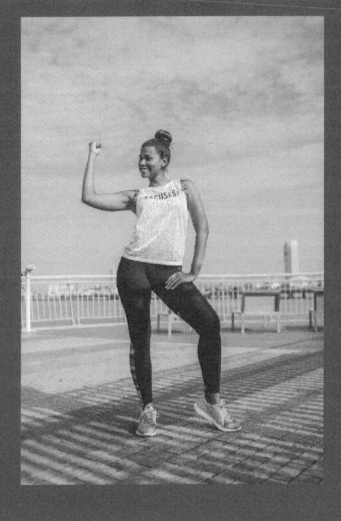

Destination Fit

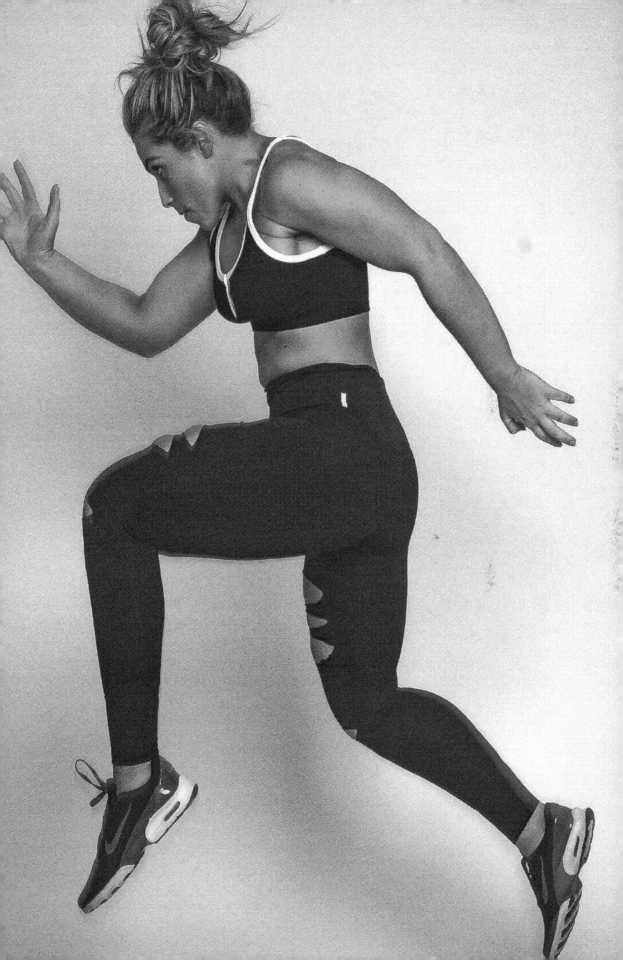

Chapter

Your fitness journey belongs to you and no one else, therefore embrace each destination!

13

Your Fitness Journey

How Do You Get Started?

For many women, the thought of beginning a fitness-training program is an exciting life changing adventure, but often, this excitement gets replaced with frustration and confusion. The feeling of frustration is often the result of not knowing where or how to start their fitness-training program. With so many books on fitness, some women are left feeling overwhelmed, confused and discouraged. Have you ever felt this way?

Have you ever felt this frustration?

Have you ever wondered how to acquire the necessary tools needed to create a fit body?

If you have, your frustration is over. I am about to take you step-by-step and teach you how to get into the best shape of your life. Are you ready? Let's take the first step!

Let the Journey Begin

The first step to getting in shape is to discover your body type. Every woman's body is unique and knowing your body type will provide you with an understanding of how your body responds to exercise and how to properly train your body in order to reach your fitness goals. Understanding your body type will hopefully help you from comparing your body to your girlfriends and other women. Let's identify your body type.

FIT JEWEL

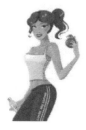

Your body is a masterpiece and you are the artist. What will your masterpiece look like?

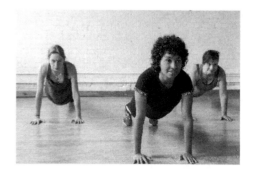

Step 1. Discover Your Body Type

Discovering your body type is an important step in creating an individualized fitness-training program to meet your individualized fitness goals. Having an understanding of your body type will help you set realistic goals and expectations and relieve you from trying to make your girlfriend's fitness program work for you.

They are three main body types, which include ectomorph (banana), mesomorph (apple or triangle) and endomorph (bell or pear). It is common for women to be a combination of two body types. Due to your individuality, it is important that you do not compare your body to other women. Your body may be smaller on top and larger on the bottom, or you may be larger on top and smaller on the bottom. Whatever your body type, you have your own unique structural foundation and your training should be tailored accordingly.

Below are descriptions of each body type and the recommended resistance and cardiovascular training. Read all descriptions and determine which is a realistic category for your body.

ECTOMORPH BODY TYPE

Body Description

Thin body structure, short torso, thin limbs and narrow feet and hands. Has difficulty putting on weight and does not carry a lot of muscle.

Unlike the mesomorph and the endomorph, the ectomorph is a person who has been skinny their entire life. It is not a result of a good diet or strict workout ethics. They are born with a superfast metabolism which allows their body to break food down at a higher rate. This gives them the "ability" to eat whatever they desire and not gain weight.

Resistance Training

The use of moderately light weights in combination with a repetition range of 12-15 can help tone the ectomorph body type. People with this body type may lack strength, therefore if strength is a goal, lifting heavier weight is required (15 pounds or more) to become stronger.

Cardiovascular Activity

Due to the high metabolism of this body type, performing an excessive amount of cardiovascular activity is not advantageous. Performing high amounts of cardio will prevent this body type from developing lean, toned muscles. Therefore performing 30-35 minutes of cardiovascular activities will help maintain lean muscle and not promote a stringy appearance and be sufficient to maintain cardiovascular health. Sufficient caloric intake is important to fuel this body type.

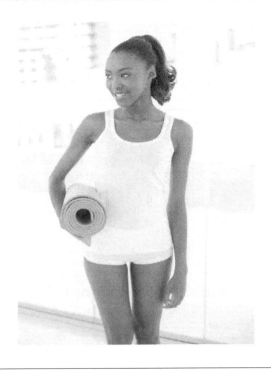

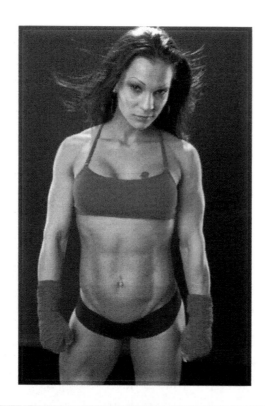

MESOMORPH BODY TYPE

Body Description

Naturally athletic, broad shoulders, narrow waist and the ability to gain muscle easily. Unlike the ectomorph, this body type doesn't have a problem gaining weight in the form of muscle or fat.

Resistance Training

Moderate to heavy weights can be used (depending on current fitness level) to maintain athletic build. A range of 8-15 repetitions with 3-4 sets per muscle group will help build dense muscle tissue without giving the bulky look. If you desire less muscle, incorporate lighter weight in conjunction with a repetition range of 15-20.

Cardiovascular Activity

Perform cardiovascular activities (running, cycling) at least 4-5 days per week for at least 45 minutes. Cardiovascular activity can be performed in an interval fashion (short bursts of high intensity activity, followed by lower intensities of recovery).

Maintenance of calorie intake is important to provide sufficient energy for training and for maintaining muscle. Prolonged sessions of high intensity cardio without sufficient calories will cause body to use muscle as fuel.

ENDOMORPH BODY TYPE

Body Description

Round, usually short in stature, carries a lot of body fat around mid- section and lower body. Slow metabolism and gains weight easily.

Resistance Training

Cardiovascular and resistance training is the key for this body type. Light to moderate weight with a repetition range of 12-15 with 3-4 sets per exercise will help tone and not build muscle. Performing activities in a circuit fashion is beneficial due to the constant state of movement throughout sets that will keep heart rate up which in return will burn more calories.

Cardiovascular Activity

Moderate to high intensity cardiovascular 45 minutes to 1 hour 4-5 days per week is recommended. Cardiovascular activities can be performed in an interval fashion (short bursts of high intensity activity, followed by lower intensities of recovery).

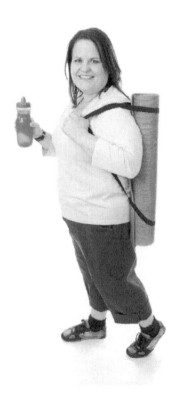

Step 2. Set Your Fitness Goals

You have discovered your body type, now it is time to learn how to set fitness training goals.

Why is it important to set goals?

Whether it is financial, marital, spiritual or physical, goal setting is an important aspect of life that keeps you focused, motivated, action-oriented and accountable. In reference to setting fitness goals, your goals should be objective, measurable, short-term, long-term and challenging - yet realistic.

Be Objective with Your Goals

Making the broad statement that you want to become fit is not concrete nor objective. You're definition of being fit needs narrowing down to a more specific or objective goal. Do you want to lose weight, gain lean muscle or improve your cardiovascular conditioning? Whatever your goal, it needs to be defined. Once your goal is defined, you can begin taking the necessary steps required to reach your desired outcome.

Measure Your Success

Goals need to be measurable. How will you determine if you are making progress if you don't know where you started? One way to determine the success of any fitness-training program is to establish a baseline of measurements. These measurements could be your body fat percentage, amount of push-ups you can perform or how quickly you can run a specific distance. Every four to six weeks you can re-access this information to determine the progress you are making towards reaching your fitness goals.

Time is of the Essence

Setting a time frame to reach your goals is imperative to reaching your destination. You can set both short-term and long-term goals that will keep you focused and accountable.

Short-term goals are goals you want to accomplish within the next 3-6 months, whereas long-term goals can be accomplished within 6 months and beyond. If you are a procrastinator, setting short-term goals is very important to keep you focused and accountable. Deciding not to establish a time frame to accomplish your goal(s) threatens your chance of reaching your desired outcome.

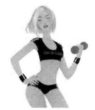

FIT JEWEL

Don't focus on your girlfriend's goals, establish your own. Your goals should be just as unique as you are!

Set Challenging Yet Realistic Goals

Finally, goals need to be challenging, yet realistic. Setting unrealistic goals perpetuates the feeling of discouragement and failure. Failure of goal attainment isn't always based on a lack of effort on your part, rather a result of setting goals that were not realistically attainable. Challenge yourself, but be realistic with your expectations.

Guidelines for Goal Setting

- Goals should be measurable.
- Goals should be challenging, yet attainable.
- Set short-term and long-term goals.
- Goals should be specific and objective.

Benefits of Setting Goals

- Greater sense of personal achievement

- Balanced life
- Increased motivation
- Improved self-confidence
- Better decision making
- Better focus
- Improved time management
- Over all self-improvement
- AND SUCCESS!

Step 3. Measure and Assess

You have discovered your body type, have learned how to set fitness goals and now it's time to discuss the importance of measurements.

Why are measurements important?

Measurements are an essential component to the success of your fitness program or weight loss program. Prior to starting any fitness or weight loss program, it is important to gather a baseline of information to determine a starting point and an ending point. How will you know if you're making progress towards your desired goal if you don't know where you started?

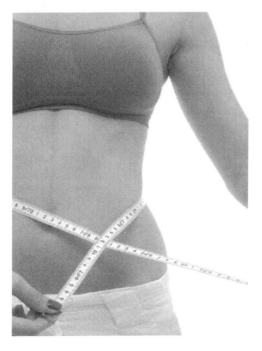

Baseline measurements can include your current weight, Body Mass Index (B.M.I), muscular endurance, flexibility and muscular strength testing. Gathering information from these sources can help you keep track of your results and every 4-6 weeks comparing your current results to your starting baseline measurements.

Below you will discover the most common methods used to gather baseline information.

Methods of Measuring Body Composition

When you hear the words body composition, what do you think? Do you know what these words mean?

In the health and fitness world, these words are thrown around like a hot dog at a baseball game. These words are familiar to personal trainers and health care providers, but they may be foreign to you.

Body composition is a term used to describe the components that make up your body, such as lean mass, fat mass and water. One primary goal of any fitness or weight loss program is to decrease fat mass and increase lean mass. Don't worry, you won't get bulky and look manly from gaining lean and toned muscle mass.

It is important to decrease fat mass and increase lean muscle tissue for many health reasons. Fat mass such as visceral fat which surrounds the internal organs has been linked to various health concerns, such as diabetes, hypertension and some forms of cancer.

Therefore, in order to make improvements in your health (and not just your appearance), you need a fitness program that focuses on gaining lean, toned muscle while at the same time losing amounts of unwanted body fat.

So how can you determine how much body fat and lean muscle mass you have?

There are several different ways that are free and painless!

I know a lot of you cringe at the thought of getting your measurements done but no worries, in the end, it will benefit your health and you will look great.

I don't want to know my numbers!

If you are one of those women who cringe at the thought of seeing measurements from your body, I want to put you at ease. These numbers don't define you; they just help to establish a starting point. I know - numbers, numbers and more numbers. You may be asking "Do I have to?" My answer is, "YES."

I promise you, the process will be done quickly and it's painless.

We are now going to discuss the three most common and inexpensive ways to get your body composition measurements done.

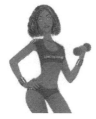

FIT JEWEL

You'll never know how far you've come, if you don't know where you started.

Fat Calipers

What is a fat caliper and how does it work?

A fat caliper is a small non-expensive prong-like tool used to measure subcutaneous (underneath skin) body fat. The tester will have you stand in an upright position with arms out to your side. He or she will ask to touch your right arm and then proceed to mark designated anatomical locations (body)

with a marker. The tester will then take their index finger and thumb and grasp at least 2 inches of your skin. The caliper will slightly grab your skin and then be released. This is a painless process that will take a few minutes to complete.

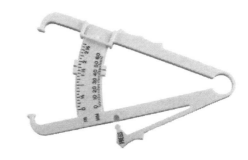

Once each spot has been located and measured, data (numbers) from the measurements are plugged into an equation to determine your percentage of body fat. Fat caliper measurements are not exact measurements, but provide you with a baseline of numbers to establish your current state of fat mass.

In order to have consistency with your measurements, have the same person administer your testing. Although each tester is required to use the same anatomical (body) locations, some testers measure differently. This difference could cause a slight variation in your numbers. You can visit your local gym or wellness center and request to have this test done for a required fee.

Below is a list of the most common anatomical locations used for measurements.

Anatomical Measuring Locations

- Triceps (back of arm)
- Supra iliac (top of hip bone)
- Sub-scapula (beneath shoulder blade)
- Biceps (middle of arm between shoulder and elbow)
- Midaxiallary- below armpit

- Subscapula-below shoulder blade
- Thigh - midway between top of hip and knee

Girth Measurements

What is a girth measurement?

A girth measurement is a measurement that records the distance around a body part. Using this method is a non-expensive and convenient way to measure your body circumference and can be done by yourself or a trained professional. Girth measurements are sometimes used as a measure of body fat, but are not a valid predictor of this, however, can be used to measure proportionality.

How are girth measurements taken?

The only tool required to take your girth measurements is a flexible measuring tape. The person administering these measurements will use specified anatomical locations. To ensure as much accuracy as possible, the person administering the test should make sure measuring tape isn't positioned too tight or too loose and the tape is placed in a horizontal position.

Having the tape too tight or too loose will not give you accurate measurements. Once data is collected, the administrator will use a formula to give you a total for each of your measurements. If you do not have someone to do your measurements for you, the process is simple enough to do the measurements on your own. If you are measuring yourself, once you gather your numbers write them down in your journal and every 4-6 weeks compare your numbers to see if they are changing. It is important to remember if you are building muscle tissue some numbers may increase. That is expected so do not be alarmed.

Where do you take your girth measurements?

There are several different places to take your measurements

- **Bust:** measure all the way around your bust and back starting at the nipple line.
- **Waist:** measure at the smallest point around your mid- section two inches above your navel.
- **Thigh:** measure at the largest part of thigh, midway between hip and knee bone.
- **Calf muscle:** measure largest part midway between knee cap and ankle.
- **Arm:** measure the largest part of arm midway between shoulder joint and elbow.
- **Hips:** measure the largest part of your buttocks, place tape on thighs and measure all the way around largest part of hips.

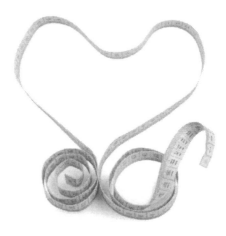

Weight Scale

Using a weight scale is a cheap and convenient way to track your weight loss or gain. You can order an inexpensive scale online or you may visit your neighborhood Wal-Mart or Walgreens to purchase a more advanced scale that is capable of recording your body fat percentage and lean muscle mass. These advanced scales are more costly, but a great investment.

Although using a weight scale is a quick and convenient way to track your weight loss or gain, if not used in moderation, this method could lead to counterproductive behaviors.

Weighing yourself too often may discourage and distract you. It is important to remember that your body changes on a daily basis, and as a result your numbers may not always be consistent. Therefore, do not depend solely on the scale to dictate your progress. Although not recommended, if you decide to weigh yourself daily, do it early in the morning at the same time on a regular basis prior to eating or drinking anything - this is your true bodyweight.

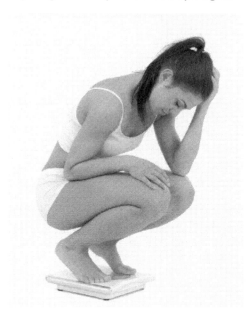

Do not weigh yourself more than once a week. Healthy weight loss is a pound to two pounds per week. If you have a considerable amount of weight to lose (100lbs or more), you may lose more in beginning but will eventually tapper off. Eventually your body will stop shedding as much body fat and you will have to

re-adjust your nutrition and fitness training program to jump-start your metabolism.

Do not allow yourself to get off track by weighing yourself every day. Instead, focus your attention on energy levels, how you feel in your clothing and mental focus.

BODY MASS INDEX Measurements

What is a BMI measurement?

BMI stands for body mass index. BMI measurements are used in many health settings to help determine body fat in relation to one's height. As with any measurement, the BMI index is not an exact science.

There are many factors such as age, muscle mass and gender that are not considered in this measurement. Someone with an athletic body may register high on the BMI scale, but in all actuality have more lean mass than fat mass. Therefore, this measurement should be used with the existing knowledge that it isn't the most accurate measurement of body fat.

Although the BMI isn't an exact measure for body fat, it is a great tool to use if you want to determine whether you are at a healthy body weight for your height or at risk for certain health concerns. High BMI's (>30) have been linked to diseases such as hypertension, high cholesterol, diabetes and obesity. Finding your BMI is a simple process that does not require expensive tools or a trained professional.

How do you calculate your BMI?

The only thing you need to calculate your BMI is a calculator and a piece of paper.

The first step in calculating your BMI is to know your current height and weight. If you do not know your current weight, find a scale and weigh yourself. If you are not aware of your height, find a measuring tape and have someone measure your height.

Follow the example below to determine your BMI by plugging in your height and weight. If you are not comfortable with numbers, you may search the World Wide Web to find a free BMI calculator to do the math for you.

Example: Amy is 150 pounds and 5 feet 8 inches (68 inches) tall. Try this one for practice and then plug in your measurements in order to calculate your own BMI.

BMI Equation: Weight (kg)/Height (m) squared

1. **Determine weight in kilograms.**

   Divide pounds by 2.2. (Dividing by 2.2 converts pounds into kilograms)

   (Ex). 150/2.2 = 68.2 kg

2. **Determine height in meters squared.**

   First, determine ht. in cm.

   (Ex). 68 inches x 2.54 = 172.72 cm.

   Next, divide ht. in cm. by 100 to get ht. in meters.

   (Ex). 172.72/100 = 1.73

   Then, square ht. in meters.

   (Ex). 1.73 x 1.73 = 2.98

3. **Divide weight in kg (68.2) by height in meters squared (2.98) = 23**

4. Go to the chart below and find whether or not Amy is at a healthy BMI. If your answer is yes, then you have calculated the right answer.

BMI Categories

BMI less than 18.5, falls within the "underweight" range.

BMI 18.5 to 24.9, it falls within the "normal" or "healthy weight" range.

BMI 25.0 to 29.9, it falls within the "overweight" range. Therefore, you may need to lose weight, especially if you have two or more of the risk factors for diseases associated with "overweight" range.

BMI 30.0 or higher falls within the "obese" range. Therefore, you should talk to your doctor or health care provider about weight loss options.

BMI >40, falls within the range of "morbid obesity" Therefore, you should talk to your doctor or health care provider about weight loss options and determine if you are healthy enough to exercise.

How Fit Are You?

For many women, being fit means weighing a certain amount on the scale and wearing a particular clothing size. Although having a healthy weight is important for health reasons, it doesn't define whether or not someone is fit. Being fit is a combination of muscular strength, muscular endurance, flexibility and cardiovascular endurance.

Bye, bye scale, hello pushups!

The only tools needed to determine your current level of fitness is a stopwatch, partner and yoga mat.

Are you ready?

One-Minute Sit-Up Test:

Purpose: This test is used to determine abdominal endurance and strength. Abdominal endurance and strength are important for core stability and back support.

A. Lay on your back with knees bent. Fingers must be interlocked behind the neck and the back of hands must touch the mat. Another person holds your ankles with hands only. If you don't have someone to hold your ankles, place your feet under a firm and stable surface such as a couch.

B. On go, you or your partner will start the stop watch and you will bring your body up and bring your elbows to touch thighs. You will lower your body and return to the ground where only the upper portion of your back touches the ground. Repeat movement for one minute and then count the number of sit-ups completed. Record your numbers.

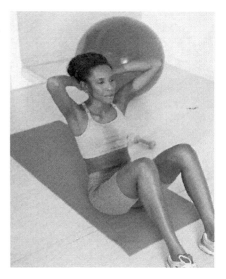

Push-Up Test (upper body strength and endurance):

Purpose: The one-minute push-up test is used to assess upper body strength and endurance.

A. Begin with body in push up position. A standard push up begins with the hands and toes touching the floor, the body and legs in a straight line, feet together, arms shoulder width apart with slight bend in elbows.

B. Keeping the back and knees straight, lower your body to a predetermined point, or until there is a 90-degree angle of the elbows, pause for a second and then return to the starting position with the arms extended without locking elbows. Repeat this action for one minute. Record your numbers.

C. If you do not have the upper body strength, perform push-ups on knees, this is considered the modified version.

3-minute Step-Up Test

Purpose: The 3-Minute Step Test measures your aerobic (cardiovascular) fitness level based on how quickly your heart rate returns to normal after exercise.

A. Before test begins, measure your resting heart rate.

Measure your resting heart rate: To do this, turn your hand over so the palm of your hand is facing upwards towards the ceiling. Locate the top of your thumb and follow your thumb until you get to the ending point of your hand. From there, using your index and middle finger, locate your radial pulse (which is located inside the hand at the base of your thumb). Don't press too hard, but gently feel for a pulse. Once you have found a pulse, set your timer and count the number of times you feel a pulse for 15 seconds and then multiply this number by 4. This is your resting pulse rate. Record your numbers.

B. From there, locate a chair or bench that is at least 12 inches high. Stand in front of the bench or chair. Start the timer and slowly step on bench/chair with one foot. Then bring other foot on bench. Use a four-step cadence, "up-up-down-down" for 3 minutes with a steady pace. At any time you feel out of breath or tired, stop for a moment in a standing position. Stop immediately on completion of 3 minutes.

C. Take pulse immediately after 3 minutes as explained in step A. Multiply the number of beats you count by 4.

D. This number represents your heart rate after exercising.

Example: 22 beats X 4 = 88 beats per minute

The quicker your heart rate drops to its resting rate, means your cardiovascular system is becoming more conditioned. In 4-6 weeks you will re-do this test and your heart rate should not get as high and you should reach your resting heart rate quicker due to your heart being more conditioned. Remember this is a starting point; you're a work in progress.

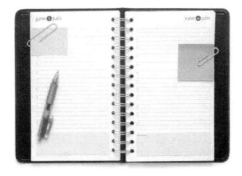

Reassess, Reassess, Reassess

Once you gather your numbers and measurements, record them and place them in your fitness journal. Four to six weeks from your original assessment date, you will want to reassess your measurements and fitness testing. You will perform the exact tests you performed above, and then compare results.

If you have noticed a positive change in numbers (ex. more strength, better cardiovascular conditioning, decreased girth measurements, BMI and Heart Rate), your fitness-training program is working and it will be time to set new fitness goals.

If you're not improving, it is recommended to re-evaluate your fitness program and motivation. During your evaluation, be honest with yourself and hold yourself accountable. Identify areas that are hindering you from reaching your goals, and from there set a realistic plan of action to reach your desired destination.

If you have not reached your goal, don't result to negative self-talk, you are working on being the best version of yourself and negative self-talk won't get you there.

Step 4. Create a Plan of Action

Let me ask you a question. Would you go on a road to trip to a particular destination without an address or directions?

Would you go on a road trip without a map or directions?

More than likely your answer is no. The same principle applies for reaching your fitness goals. It is harder to reach your destination without direction. Therefore once you have your measurements and fitness assessment numbers recorded, it's time create a plan of attack to reach your desired fitness goals.

If your goal is to do more push-ups within a minute and build upper body strength, then a plan of action to build upper body strength is required. If you desire better cardiovascular conditioning, a cardiovascular program needs to be designed.

Whatever your goals, your plan of action needs to create the right steps to help you reach your destination.

How do you create a plan of action? Let's find out.

FIT JEWEL

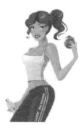

Having no plan of action to get fit will leave you frustrated and distracted. Create a plan and work your plan, you're worth it!

Create Your Plan of Attack

The first step in creating your plan of action is to find physical activities and exercise that you enjoy. If you enjoy something, you are more likely to stick with it and reach your goals easier. Working out should be an exciting time to focus on yourself and not feel tortured during the process. Therefore, it is essential to find something you enjoy doing. Many gyms offer group fitness classes including kickboxing, Zumba, spin and boot camps. Try each one of these classes to determine which classes you enjoy most. Choose classes that are fun and are most beneficial to help you reach your fitness goal.

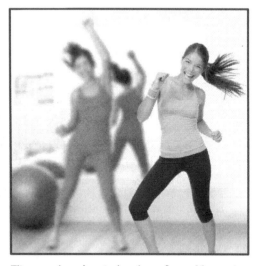

Fitness is about having fun. Move to your own beat. If you like to dance, just dance!

If you decide group fitness classes work for you, alternate classes to avoid overuse injuries and boredom. Overuse injuries are the result of performing the same movement patterns on a consistent basis. Constant movement patterns stress the same muscles and joints and can lead to chronic (long-term) or acute (short-term) injuries. In addition to possible overuse injuries, attending the same classes will eventually cause your body to hit a plateau and lead to limited changes in your body and cardiovascular conditioning levels.

Determine How Many Days to Exercise

Once you determine which activities you enjoy, it's time to realistically determine how many days per week you are willing to dedicate to these activities. You know your commitments more than anyone else, therefore don't commit to more days than you can handle with your current lifestyle. If you can only do three days a week, some physical activity is better than no exercise at all. If you can't get all three days in, do what you can and don't fall into the "all or none" philosophy once you set your days of the week to exercise.

What is the "all or none" philosophy?

The "all or none" philosophy is a belief that if you miss one session of your planned activity during the week than there is no point of going for the entire week. This is a negative philosophy and mentality that can keep you from reaching your fitness goal(s). Therefore, I will once again reiterate, be realistic about the amount of days you can commit to your fitness program and some exercise is better than no exercise.

Keep Moving - It's Just Life!

If we lived in the perfect world, we could spend as much time as we wanted dedicated to getting fit, but unfortunately the world and our lives aren't perfect and we have to be flexible with getting enough physical activity in.

We get busy, emergencies and unexpected events happen, things come up that are out of our control and we sometimes get thrown off schedule, but when this happens, keep going and adapt.

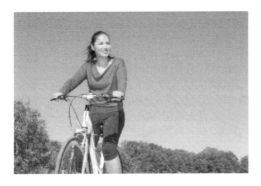

Five Tips to Keep Your Body Moving When Life Happens

1. If you can't make it to your normal scheduled class, try another class. If you normally go to a 6:00 pm class and you're running late, try a 6:30 pm class. If there isn't one available, get creative in the gym and try a new piece of cardio equipment or resistance training machine. Do not leave the gym without doing something healthy for yourself.

2. Can't make it to the gym? Go for a walk. You don't have to attend the gym to get fit. If you can't make it on a particular day, go for a walk. Walking is a great way to relieve stress and clear your mind.

3. Keep an extra set of gym clothes and shoes in your car. If you have to go back home to get your workout clothes, more than likely you're not going back to the gym. Therefore, always keep an extra set of gym clothes and shoes in your trunk. Consider this your emergency gym kit.

4. You wake up late - make the most of the time you have. If you don't wake up when the alarm goes off and all you have is 10 minutes to exercise, do something. Keep in mind doing 10 minutes of some exercise is better than no exercise at all.

5. Your boss tells you that you have to work later than planned. If you have to work longer than expected and you're going to miss your workout, take a brisk walk around your office building. If you have stair cases in your building, take the stairs for an allotted period of time. Don't panic, life happens, just keep moving.

Step 5. Determine Your Motivation

What's Your Motivation?

The last step in beginning your fitness journey is to discover your motivation. Discovering your motivation may help you become more consistent with your fitness training program.

In order to discover how you are motivated, it's important to identify your motivation style.

Are you intrinsically or extrinsically motivated?

Someone who is intrinsically motivated is self-motivated and reaches goals for self-gratification and not external rewards. Intrinsically motivated people are driven by something within themselves and do not need anyone to motivate them. They set goals for themselves and are motivated to accomplish those goals without any external reward or a required cheering squad.

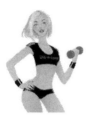

FIT JEWEL

What makes you want to move? Discover it and run with it!

Tips for Extrinsically Motivated People

- Reward yourself with non-food related items when you met certain goals.

- Place a picture of what you want to look like on your fridge and in your training journal - this may help provide you with visual motivation.

- When you reach a goal, share it with someone in your support team. Sharing your success will help keep you motivated.

Then there are those who are extrinsically motivated. Extrinsically motivated people are individuals who need an external force (such as rewards or praise from other people) to motivate them. They need consistent feedback and support to feel they are doing well and without support, they are less likely to complete the task they have started. Neither one of these motivational styles are wrong, we are individuals and are driven by different motivating factors.

If you are more geared towards being extrinsically motivated, below are a few tips for you.

Steady But Gradual Progress

If you're feeling overwhelmed by all the steps you have just learned, exhale for a moment and tell yourself to focus on the process and not the outcome. Allow yourself the freedom to embrace this process without expectations of time. Your fitness journey is a jog and not a sprint, and I am confident that you will reach your destination if you give yourself time.

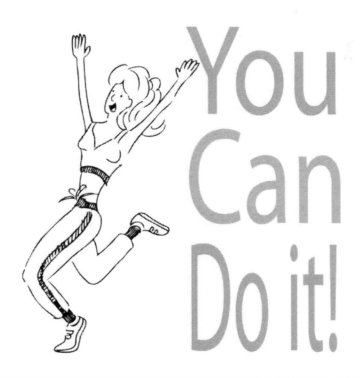

Chapter

Learn these principles and transform your body!

14

Resistance Training 101

Before You Begin

Before you make the decision to pick up a dumbbell or workout on a weight machine, it is important to understand a few key lifting techniques and training methods. These techniques and training methods will help you avoid injury and provide you with information to navigate through the Iron Palace (gym) with more confidence.

Lifting Techniques

Whenever you perform an exercise (either on a machine or with free weights) there are two primary phases of movements. These phases of movement include an eccentric and concentric phase.

The concentric phase of a movement occurs when the muscle contracts or shortens. If you were executing a bicep curl, curling the weight up is the concentric phase of the movement.

The opposite, or opposing movement, is called the eccentric movement. The eccentric phase of movement involves lengthening or releasing the weight back to the starting position. If you were performing a dumbbell bicep curl, and released your hand and allow the dumbbell to move downward away from your body, this would be the eccentric phase.

Each phase of movement challenges the muscles from a different level of difficulty, and one cannot be completed without the other. Therefore, it is important to only lift an amount of weight you can control during each phase of the movement. Never jeopardize form to lift heavier weight.

If an amount of weight is too heavy, choose a lighter weight. Once again I will reiterate, do not sacrifice form in order to lift a heavier amount of weight. Choosing to lift heavy weight in which you can't lift properly through both phases of movement can result in acute and permanent injuries.

Lifting Posture Standing

While performing any lifting movement in a standing position, feet are to be positioned slightly apart with knees slightly bent. Core or abdominals are held in tight, with shoulder blades back and chest up. Never round your back and be aware of your posture at all times.

Posture on Machines

Each machine is created to operate in a fixed range of motion meaning you can only move the machine in a predetermined movement pattern. This is beneficial in many ways but proper posture is still required while using machines. Proper posture involves controlled movements and keeping core engaged at all times throughout the exercise.

Proper Breathing

Proper breathing consists of inhaling at the starting phase of the movement, before the beginning of the lift (concentric phase), and exhaling during the release of the weight (eccentric phase). Holding your breath while lifting can cause dizziness and create a lack of oxygen to working muscles.

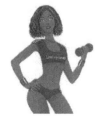

FIT JEWEL

You're truly an iron sister at heart, you just don't know it yet!

Training Methods

We have discovered proper lifting techniques, now it's time to learn different resistance training methods. The following resistance training methods are the most common and most applicable.

Split Training

Split training is a term used to identify how each muscle group is divided and trained. Using the split training method ensures each muscle group is trained on a consistent basis, in order to avoid muscular imbalances and muscular injuries from under and overdeveloped muscles.

How do you create a split training routine that is right for you?

In order to create your individualized split, determine how many days a week you can dedicate to resistance training. Once you have completed this task, decide which muscle groups you want to train together or by themselves (ex. Biceps and Triceps, Back and Chest). Some research suggests training your muscles in a push/pull fashion, but you make the decision. This method is believed to create muscular balances if done properly.

Training in a push/pull fashion involves training muscles that allow you to perform pushing and pulling movements within the same training session. Doing a push up is considered a pushing movement (which uses your chest muscles), followed by seated dumbbells rows (which is a pulling movement) which works the back muscles.

Split training is designed based on individual preference, and your split may not mirror your girlfriends. Once you create your split schedule, it does not have to be set in stone. Changing the muscle groups and the days you train them are beneficial both mentally and physically.

Possible Disadvantage of the Split Training Method

Although split training is a great training method, it is important to consider your current level of fitness before you create your split training routine.

Spilt training typically focuses on training one or two body parts per training session. Typically, the volume or the number of sets and repetitions you perform using this training method places more stress on your muscles. Placing a great amount of stress on untrained muscles can lead to excessive soreness and injuries. Therefore, if you are not at a training level where you can perform split training, full body training may be more advantageous for you.

Advantages of Split Training

A benefit of split training for seasoned lifters is the ability to train a weak muscle group(s). With this method of training, you can focus on that particular group during your training session and perform more sets which can assist in strengthening your weaker muscle groups.

Example of Split Training

Monday:	Biceps/Triceps/Abs
Tuesday:	Chest/Back
Wednesday:	Off
Thursday:	Shoulders/Abs
Friday:	Legs/Abs
Saturday:	Off

Full Body Training

As the name states, full body training is a method that targets each major muscle group within one training session. Full body training is a great method for beginners and for individuals who do not have enough time to devote to a split training regimen.

Full body training targets each muscle group, but it doesn't stress each individual muscle group as efficiently as split training. When you are doing a full body training session, you are typically performing one or two exercises per muscle group. This will help you tone, but in order to have continual muscle growth, you will eventually need to stress each muscle group beyond full body training.

Example of Full Body Training

2 sets per exercise, 12-15 repetitions

	Set 1	Set 2
Legs	Lunges	Squats
Biceps	Bicep Curls	Hammer Curls
Triceps	Triceps Extensions	Triceps Kickbacks
Shoulders	Lateral Shoulder Raises	Front Shoulder Raises
Back	One-arm Rows	Seated Rows
Abs	Crunches	Leg Lifts

Super Setting

Super setting requires performing one exercise for a primary muscle group, followed immediately by performing an exercise for its opposing muscle group. Super setting keeps your muscles in balance due to the consistency of training both sides of your muscle group.

Super setting will cut back on gym time and allow the body to maintain balance within each muscle group.

Example of Super Setting

Biceps/Triceps (bicep curls followed immediately by triceps extensions)

Back/Chest (lat pull downs, followed immediately by pushups)

Quads/Hamstrings (leg extensions, followed immediately by hamstring curls)

Giant Set

Performing a giant set requires choosing a particular muscle group and choosing 4-5 different exercises for that particular group.

After choosing your exercises, perform each exercise in a circuit fashion, moving from one exercise to another without rest until the set is complete.

Create your giant set based on your current fitness level. You can begin with 2-3 different exercises, and then progressively increase the amount of exercises as you become stronger and better conditioned.

Example of a Giant Set

Muscle Group: Shoulders

Lateral shoulder raises	10 repetitions
Front shoulder raises	10 repetitions
Seated shoulder press	10 repetitions
Rear deltoid raises	10 repetitions

Circuit Training

Circuit training involves performing a group of exercises in a continuous fashion, and not reaching a stopping point until each exercise is completed.

Circuit training is believed to be an effective training method for people who are short on time and desire more cardiovascular conditioning.

Cardiovascular conditioning is a result of a continually elevated heart rate throughout the circuit.

Example of Circuit Training

Remember to perform each exercise in a continual fashion before you reach a state of rest.

Stationary lunges	12 repetitions
Standing bicep curls	12 repetitions
Triceps kickbacks	12 repetitions
Standing shoulder press	12 repetitions
Modified pushups	8-10 repetitions
Crunches	12 repetitions

Interval Training

Interval training involves performing short periods of high intensity exercise followed immediately by the same activity at a lower intensity.

Studies show interval training burns more calories than regular steady state (performing exercise at same pace over a period of time) physical activities.

Intervals can be created during any activity.

Example of Interval Training

An example of interval training would be sprinting on the treadmill at a 6.9 speed for 30 seconds followed by jogging at a speed of 4.0 for one minute. Repeat interval five times)

Determine Your Sets, Repetitions and Weight

One of the most common questions women have when it comes to resistance training is, "How much weight should I lift in order to reach my goals?"

The amount of weight you lift is based on your fitness goals. If you desire to build toned, lean muscles, you will perform exercises with light weight (5-15 pounds) within a repetition range of 15-20 repetitions while performing at least three sets of each exercise.

If your goal is to build an athletic body with more dense muscle tissue, you will lift heavier weight (15 pounds or more)

within a range of 8-15 repetitions performing at least 4-5 sets of each exercise.

As a rule of thumb, the heavier weight you use, the fewer repetitions you will perform. This builds strength and muscle density.

The lighter weight you use, the higher repetitions you will perform. This will create lean, toned muscles.

Wait I Still Have Questions!

Walking into a room full of men with bulging biceps can leave you doubting the choice you have made to start a resistance training program, but equipping yourself with the proper armor before you enter the Iron Palace will give you more confidence and the ability to freely navigate your way through.

Entering the Iron Palace may seem intimidating right now, but in order to provide you with more tools, below you will discover answers to the most frequently asked questions from women regarding resistance and cardiovascular training. Knowing the answers to these questions may help you feel more confident.

FAQs Regarding Resistance and Cardiovascular Training

> Q.
>
> HOW MANY DAYS A WEEK SHOULD I LIFT?

A.

It is recommended that beginners start with 2-3 days per week performing total body workouts or using machines. The beginning of your fitness training program should be gradual, with an emphasis on technique or lifting form. Training too frequently or intensely at this stage of your fitness-training program could lead to injuries and early burn out.

Intermediate and advanced trainees can train 4-5 days per week, allowing at least 48 hours of rest per muscle group. If you are in a training rut, revamp your entire fitness training program by overloading your body with more repetitions, heavier weight, different exercises and less rest time in between sets.

A rule of thumb - if you have been using the same fitness training program for more than 6 weeks, it is time to update your program.

Q.

MACHINES OR FREE WEIGHTS?

A.

Both. Using a combination of machines and free weights can assist you in reaching your fitness goals.

Machines

Machines are great for beginners, they are easy to operate and provide step-by-step instructions. Most machines provide pictorials to identify which muscle groups are used during the execution of the movement. Machines are created to move in a fixed range of motion that prevents improper form and this is beneficial to individuals who aren't experienced with resistance training. Using machines does not require a high level of coordination, balance or strength for beginners.

Free Weights

Using free weights requires proper knowledge of form in order to execute each desired exercise. Using free weights also requires balance, coordination and core strength. Free weights engage more muscular activity

than using machines and can challenge the body in a different manner than machines. More muscle engagement means more calories burned. More calories burned means a more lean and toned body.

Q.

HOW MUCH WEIGHT SHOULD I LIFT?

A.

Beginners

Beginners are recommended to find an amount of weight that will allow them to perform 12-15 repetitions safely throughout an entire range of movement. When reaching the 15th repetition if the weight is still challenging to lift, stay with that amount of weight. Once you reach a point where the weight is no longer challenging, make small increases in weight. You can progress from 5 lbs. to 8 lbs. then to 10 lbs. This process is known as progressive resistance training.

Intermediate and Advanced Trainees

Select an amount of weight heavy enough that will allow you to execute 8-15 repetitions with proper form. If you reach your 15th repetition and the weight is not challenging, increase the weight by 5 lbs.

Q.

HOW MANY REPETITIONS DO I PERFORM?

A.

The number of repetitions performed for any exercise is determined by your fitness goals.

- 2-3 repetitions

- Heavy weight

- This will help athletes develop power and explosiveness.

For Muscular Strength

- 8-15 repetitions

- Moderate to heavy weight

- This will help build lean and dense muscle tissue.

For Muscular Endurance

- 15- 20 repetitions

- Light weight

- This will help tone lean muscles.

Q.

HOW MUCH CARDIO SHOULD I DO?

A.

Cardiovascular activity should be a part of every person's fitness training program, but shouldn't be the only method used to get fit. Cardiovascular activities not only burn body fat, they keep your heart (the most important muscle in your body) in shape, but they don't build lean muscles.

According to The American College of Sports Medicine and the American Heart Association, perform at least 60 minutes of moderate- to vigorous physical activity most days of the week.

However, the specific amount of cardio you need varies from person to person and depends on the following factors:

- Daily caloric intake

- Exercise intensity and frequency

- Your metabolic rate (rate of substance breakdown)

- Your current fitness level (sedentary individuals will require a gradual increase in cardiovascular activities)

- Your body fat percentage

- Your current weight

- Your fitness goals

Beginners

Perform at least 25-30 minutes of light-to-moderate intensity cardiovascular activities most days of the week. Gradually progress where you can perform 35-45 minutes of continuous cardiovascular activities as your heart and lungs become more conditioned.

Intermediate and Advanced

Perform at least 40 minutes to 1 hour, including intervals.

Q.

WHAT IS A HEART RATE?

A.

Heart rate is the number of beats the heart takes within one minute. There is a direct correlation between heart rate and workload (work performed). As workload or intensity increases, heart rate will increase. In order to keep track of your heart rate, you may purchase a heart rate monitor. Wearing a heart rate monitor will help gauge your intensity levels at all times.

Q.

HOW DO I FIND MY PULSE RATE TO
DETERMINE HOW INTENSE I AM
EXERCISING?

A.

You can determine your pulse rate by using your radial pulse (arm).

In order to locate your radial pulse, turn your hand over with thumb turned in an outward position. Start at tip of thumb and go all the way to the base of your thumb and move about half an inch from base of thumb using index and middle fingers and search for a pulse.

Once pulse is located, count the number of heart beats for 10 seconds. Multiply this number by six. This number will give you your heart rate.

Setting a target heart rate will give you an intensity level to reach for while exercising.

Know Your Numbers

The table below shows estimated target heart rates for different ages. In the age category closest to yours, read across to find your target heart rate. Your maximum heart rate is about 220 minus your age. The figures are averages, so use them as general guidelines.

Age	Target HR Zone, 50-85%	Average Maximum Heart Rate, 100%
20 years	100-170 beats per minute	200 beats per minute
30 years	95-162 beats per minute	190 beats per minute
35 years	93-157 beats per minute	185 beats per minute
40 years	90-153 beats per minute	180 beats per minute
45 years	88-149 beats per minute	175 beats per minute
50 years	85-145 beats per minute	170 beats per minute
55 years	83-140 beats per minute	165 beats per minute
60 years	80-136 beats per minute	160 beats per minute
65 years	78-132 beats per minute	155 beats per minute
70 years	75-128 beats per minute	150 beats per minute

A.

If you are training to become powerful, power moves are performed first in your workout program. Power moves require lifting heavy amounts of weight that fatigue your neuromuscular system and should not be performed when you are fatigued. Lifting heavy amounts of weight when you are fatigued can lead to permanent injuries, therefore all power moves should occur at the beginning of your fitness routine (ex. Plyometrics)

Next, you will want to perform exercises that require the use of larger muscles (legs, chest, back) or multi-joint exercises. These exercises require more energy to perform, therefore should be done before performing single-joint exercises which require less effort.

Last to be performed are smaller or single-joint exercises (shoulders, triceps, biceps). To avoid fatigue, do not train smaller muscles first. Training your smaller muscle groups first will cause you to fatigue quicker and lead to a less-than-optimal training session for your larger muscle groups.

Q.

HOW MUCH REST TIME SHOULD I
TAKE IN BETWEEN SETS?

A.

The amount of rest time taken in between sets is determined by the amount of weight used and the intensity level at which you perform the exercise. Performing powerful and explosive movements may require 3-5 minutes of rest. This amount of rest time is needed to produce more energy and allows your neurological system time to recuperate.

For lower intensity exercises, rest for 30-90 seconds and no longer.

Q.

HOW MUCH REST TIME SHOULD I
TAKE OFF BETWEEN WORKOUT
SESSIONS?

A.

Resistance training involves breaking down muscle fibers (muscle tissue) that result in muscular soreness referred to as D.O.M.S. (Delayed Onset Muscle Soreness). The body naturally repairs these micro tears during rest. Therefore, not getting the proper amount of rest can lead to overtraining, diminishes in strength and a weakened immune system and fatigue.

Therefore, it is recommended to allow at least 48 hours of rest time between training of each muscle group. If you are afraid to take a complete day off, you may take part in activities called active rest. During active rest, you are performing more leisure-based activities such as walking the dog, gardening or maybe going for a casual walk.

Below are signs of training burnout and overtraining. Familiarize yourself with these signs and be mindful that more isn't always better!

Signs of Burnout or Overtraining

- Weakened immune system (more susceptible to infections)
- Decrease in motivation
- Excessive muscle soreness
- Irritability
- Decreases in strength
- Easily distracted

A.

No, muscle and fat are two separate types of tissue. One cannot convert into the other.

When muscle tissue is not stressed by lifting adequate amounts of weight (resistance), the muscles atrophy (become smaller).

When a person gains fat weight, it is not a result of muscle tissue turning into fat; it is a result of an increase in size of their fat cells.

Q.

SHOULD I DO CARDIO OR WEIGHTS?

A.

In order to create a strong, lean and toned physique you need to incorporate both.

To all of my resistance training enthusiasts, resistance training is great for building lean muscle tissue, but without cardiovascular activity, that six pack you have been working so hard to create may not be seen. Body fat can threaten to hide your hard-earned muscle and one of the ways you can show off what you have worked hard for is to incorporate cardiovascular activities into your regular fitness training sessions along with clean eating.

To my cardio queens, if the only thing you do is cardio, I want to encourage you to step into the Iron Palace and begin a resistance training program. Cardiovascular activities will change your size, but it will not change the shape of your body. Resistance training will help build a toned, calorie-burning machine. Muscle tissue is a dense, active tissue that burns calories even at the state of rest.

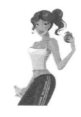

FIT JEWEL

More Muscles = More Calories

Resistance Training Principles and Terminology

Principle of Individual Differences - Everyone has a different genetic makeup and different training needs. Your fitness training program needs to be designed around your individuality. Your friend's training program may not work for you.

Principle of Adaptation - The body is a dynamic creation that changes when constant external (resistance training/weights) forces are applied. In order for your body to grow, continue to challenge your body with more repetitions, sets and volume of training.

Principle of Specificity - The only way to master a particular exercise or skill is to execute that particular exercise or skill on a regular basis. Specificity training is a very big principle in the athletic world. In order for a swimmer to become better at swimming, he/she has to swim. If you want to become great at a particular exercise, perform that exercise on a regular basis and your body will eventually adapt.

Principle of Progression - Placing too much stress or load on your body in a short period of time can lead to injuries. Therefore, gradually increase the amount of weight and intensity of each exercise you perform. Doing this will prevent excessive soreness, over training and mental burnout.

Principle of Use/Disuse - It is a cliché, but it is true. "If you don't use it, you lose it." When muscles are under consistent tension or stress, they adapt and grow. This process is called hypertrophy.

When muscles are not stressed, they become smaller and weaker. A process called atrophy. If you incorporate a resistance training program for a period of time, then stop for a longer period of time, your muscles will atrophy (become smaller). No stress means no growth.

Principle of Overload - Once the body adapts to a stress or load, it has to be challenged with more stress or load. Continuing to perform the same exercises, sets, repetitions and rest time does not challenge the body enough to force it to change. You have to overload your body and there is no way around this principle.

Abduction - movement away from the midline of the body (ex. doing seated abductions on a machine). In this exercise, you bring your legs from an inward position to an outward position.

Adduction – movement towards the midline of the body.(ex. doing seated adductions on a machine). In this exercise, you bring your legs from an outward position to an inward position.

Atrophy - loss of muscle due to lack of training stimulus.

Cardiovascular - pertains to your heart, veins and arteries.

Concentric - upward or contraction phase of a movement/muscle shortens (muscle contracts).

Dorsi Flexion - pointing toes upward towards the ceiling.

Eccentric - downward or negative phase of a movement/muscle lengthens (muscle relaxes).

Elbow extension - movement resulting in an increase of the elbow joint (triceps extension) of the body. These planes of motion allow the body to move in a certain direction and help identify movements of particular joints.

Elbow flexion - movement resulting in a decrease of the elbow joint (performing a bicep curl).

Extension - increases the angle of a joint (performing leg extensions is an example of knee extension).

Flexibility - range of motion around a joint.

Flexion - decreases the angle of a joint (oerforming a bicep curls is an example of elbow flexion).

Hyperextend - to go beyond a point or distance.

Hypertrophy - muscular growth due to training stimulus.

Lateral - side movement (ex. lateral shoulder raises).

Muscular Endurance - the ability to continually exert force against a resistance.

Maximum heart rate - the highest number of times your heart beats in one minute.

Muscular Strength - the ability to exert a maximal amount of force against resistance.

Plantar Flexion - pointing toes downward.

Primary muscle - intended targeted muscle you want to train (when performing bicep curls, primary muscle is the bicep).

Respiratory - pertains to your lungs.

Repetition - repeated movement of a particular exercise.

Rotation - side-to-side or left-to-right movement of the trunk (top part of body) (ex. performing Russian Twists) or neck.

Set - designated amount of repetitions.

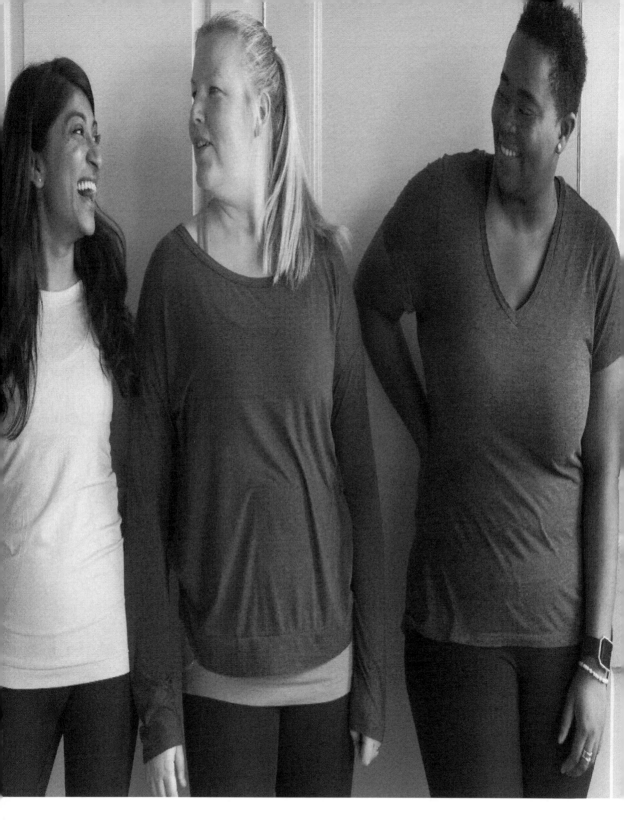

*Talking is great,
but pushing your body
to its limits is better.
When it's time to train,
it's time to train!*

15

Social Hour is Over

This Isn't Club Talk

Attending the gym and being around like-minded fitness enthusiasts can help you reach your fitness goals and possibly lead you to making lifetime friendships. This can be an exciting time for you, but working out at the gym can also be a place where you can get distracted from reaching your goals.

Distracted, who me?

As women, many of us have one thing in common, we love to socialize. Yes, many of us are social butterflies, and this can be a great thing at the right time and right place, but it is not social hour when you walk through the gym doors. You are there to train and focus on your fitness goals.

Does this mean that you have to be unfriendly and non-sociable? Not at all, but it does mean that 90 percent of your time shouldn't be spent talking. Talking and not working out will prevent you from reaching your fitness goals. If you enjoy chatting, have your talks during your cool down and stretching.

Before we continue, let me share a pet peeve of mine.

If you are new to the gym, you may not be able to relate to this, but if you're a "gymette," you will know exactly what I mean. Let me paint the picture for you.

Please Don't Distract Me!

It has been a long day at work and all you can think about is getting to the gym and having a grueling workout. OK, maybe you don't enjoy the grueling aspect of training, but follow me anyway. You rush to the gym and can't wait for some alone time.

You change into your training gear and are ready to train. You walk out into the Iron Palace and you begin your warm up. You have your music on the right song and you are starting to feel your body's core temperature increase. Ten minutes of a general warm up and you are ready to attack the IRON.

You get your gloves on and all you can think about is the feeling of iron held in your hands. You scope out your weapon of mass destruction and head in that direction. On the way there you have the eye of the tiger and all of a sudden someone stops and says "Hi, how are you?" You do not want to lose your focus and at the same time, you don't want to be rude. You say, "I'm great thanks." Another question comes. "So how is work?" You think, "Oh no, if I do not walk away more questions are going to follow."

Sure enough, you try to walk off and the person keeps talking. You are cooling down and someone has taken the equipment you wanted to use. Can you say frustrated? If you are laughing right about now, you know exactly what I am talking about.

The gym is a great place to meet people, but keep in mind - it isn't social hour when you are there. It's great to talk, but make your conversations polite and brief. Don't spend the majority of your time talking with friends or associates. If you do, you are losing time that could be invested in you transforming your body. How can you build a fit body if you spend the majority of your time talking?

A rule of thumb to keep in mind is - time spent in the gym does not automatically mean time spent on training. I frequently meet women who share that their fitness program just isn't working. When I ask them if they are in the gym for social hour or to train, many of the responses correspond with the latter.

If you are talking more than you're working, more than likely your mind is not focused on exercising. Therefore, here's your new mantra - "When it's time to train, it's time to train." Save the talking for cardio time.

Avoid Wasting Gym Time

Talk during rest time: It is great having friends at the gym, but keep in mind you are there to train and not have social hour. Talk during your rest time between sets, but stay focused on why you're there.

Plan ahead of time: Have a plan of action before you hit the gym. Know which muscle(s) you are going to train and what exercises you are going to do before you arrive. Having a plan of attack will keep you from wondering around not sure of what to do.

Don't wait around: If a machine you want is occupied, politely ask the individual when they are going to be finished. Do not waste time waiting for a particular machine. Do another exercise and come back at a later time.

Perform exercises in a circuit fashion: A circuit involves choosing at least four different exercises for the entire body, and performing one exercise then immediately performing another without reaching a state of rest until all exercises are complete. Training in this fashion will keep your heart rate up and decrease gym time.

Double check your gym bag: Before leaving home, double check your gym bag to make sure you have socks, gym shoes, training clothes and hair ties. This will help you from having to go back home or stop at the store to purchase these items. This saves time and money.

Bring your own water: Have enough water to avoid frequent trips to the water fountain. Carry a large container to hold water instead of little 16 oz bottles that require many refills.

Fuel up: Eat a source of protein and complex carbohydrate at least one hour before your workout. Not having enough fuel can hinder your workout and prevent you from fully exerting yourself.

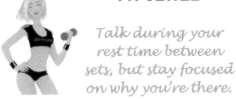

FIT JEWEL

Talk during your rest time between sets, but stay focused on why you're there.

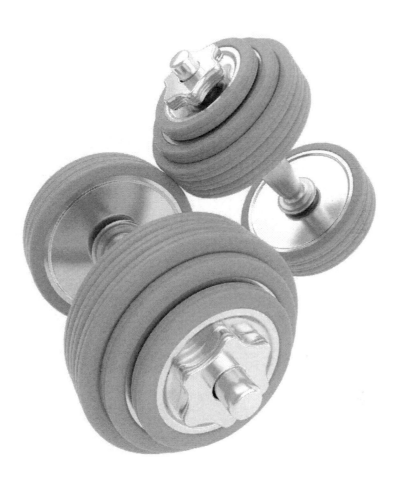

Chapter

Fitness etiquette, please. Don't forget the unspoken RULES!

16

Fit Girl's Gym Etiquette

Gym Etiquette 101

If you are newcomer to the gym, this class will be new to you. If you are a seasoned veteran, this will be a refresher course.

After spending many years in the gym, you become aware of what is acceptable and what is not. There are spoken and unspoken rules at the gym and now that you are going to be a part of this culture, it is important that you learn proper gym etiquette. The rules are as follows:

Rule 1: Don't sit in sauna without clothes

We are all women, but there is something very awkward about having someone in the nude right in front of you doing things that most people would consider private. Being comfortable in your own skin is great, but be aware there are other people who may not feel comfortable with you walking around in the nude. Embrace your body, but please put a towel on.

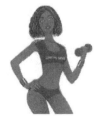

FIT JEWEL

There are spoken and unspoken rules at the gym - it's important to learn gym etiquette!

Rule 2: Don't use bathroom stalls to change clothes

The bathroom should be used just for what is has been created for. If you are uncomfortable changing in front of other people it's understandable, but please don't change in the bathroom. Doing this holds the line up when other people need to use the restroom. Please be considerate and go into the shower area or other private designated area and change. Normally there is more space in these areas, and you will not hold up the restrooms.

Rule 3: No perfume overload

There is a time and place for everything, but wearing heavy amounts of perfume to the gym is definitely not the right time or place. Instead of using heavy perfumes that may affect other people, try a light body spray.

Rule 4: No machine hoarding

Depending on the time of day, the gym can become overly crowded. If this is the case, you may have to share equipment with other people. If this happens, be open and willing to share. If you are working on a machine and taking a rest, allow someone else to use the machine during your rest time. Be friendly and respectful to everyone and if you are not using a machine, do not sit and talk on the machine. This hinders other people from using the machine.

Rule 5: Do not interrupt

It is an unspoken rule, but a very important one. Do not interrupt someone during a set. If someone is in the middle of lifting weights or performing an exercise, wait until they are done before you interrupt them. It is rude and can break someone's focus if you speak to them while they are executing a movement. If you need to ask a question, wait until that person has completed with their set. If they are not finished, do not stand and wait. Walk away and come back when they are finished.

Rule 6: No cell phone on gym floor

Cell phones can be a huge distraction to you and others. Talking on the phone while working out can be dangerous and annoying to others around you. If you need to talk, find a quiet place in the gym to excuse yourself. Some gyms do not allow members to talk on cell

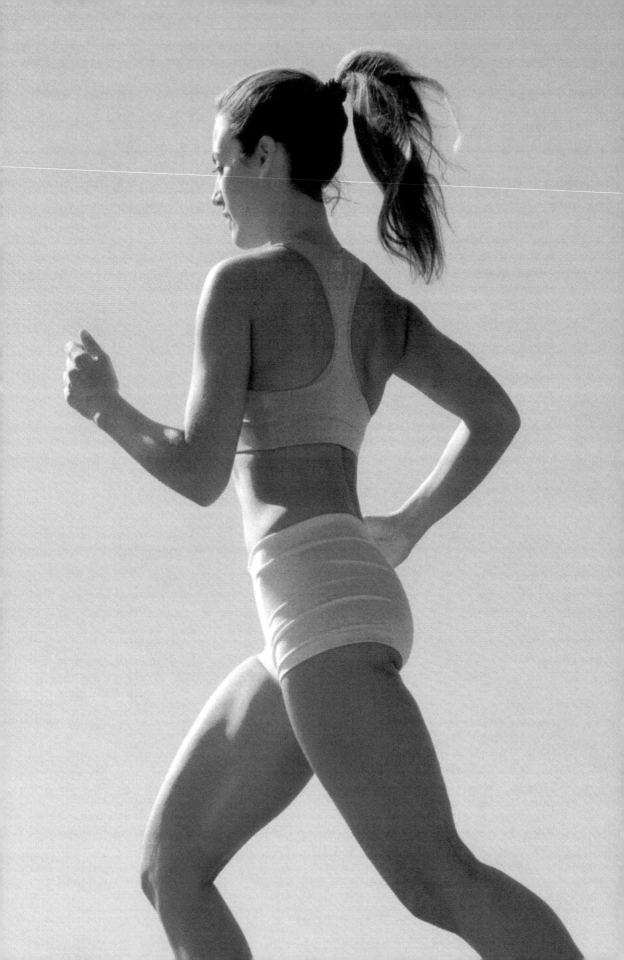

Chapter

Good-bye long hours of cardio, hello interval training!

17

Cardio Fit

Are You the Queen of Cardio?

Do you often find yourself doing hour-long cardio sessions with the hope of losing weight?

For many women, performing endless hours of cardio has become the solution to weight loss and getting into shape. Although cardio can assist you in losing weight, doing endless hours of cardio will not ultimately get your body into the best shape.

You may have been taught that this is the only way to reach your fitness and weight loss goals, but I would like to share a better way to help you reap more benefits from doing less cardio.

How does that sound?

Do Less and Reap More

Although steady state (exercising at same intensity level for a period of time) cardio has its benefits, interval training can be more beneficial and require less time.

Studies have shown that performing 15-20 minutes of interval training can burn more calories than performing 40-45 minutes of steady state cardio if done at the appropriate intensity level. Therefore, why spend endless hours doing steady state cardio, when you can spend less time and gain more results by doing interval training?

Interval What?

What is interval training?

Interval training consists of performing short bursts of high intensity activity followed by short periods of lower intensity activity. You can create an interval on any piece of cardio equipment, with running or walking.

An example of a jog/sprint interval could consist of sprinting to a certain landmark (such as a mail box) and then jogging to another land mark (such as a stop sign).

The intensity of your high bursts is based on your current level of fitness and as with any physical activity, interval training should be done in moderation and safely. Interval training requires higher bursts of movements, and if done too fast for beginners could result in injuries.

FIT JEWEL

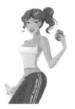

Doing endless hours of cardio will not ultimately get your body into the best shape.

Therefore, it is recommended beginners perform intervals 1-2 times per week in the beginning of your fitness program and increase the frequency as your cardiovascular condition improves.

For individuals who are intermediate or advanced, perform intervals 3-4 days per week allowing yourself at least 48 hours of rest per week. Too much of any good thing is bad for you.

How Do You Create an Interval?

Determine your current fitness level and cardiovascular conditioning (beginner, intermediate or advanced).

Determine how much cardio you desire to perform.

Choose a machine(s), or decide if you want to perform walking or running intervals.

Based on your fitness level, create an interval for a desired amount of time.

The amount of time you rest is based on the intensity of activity (e.g., you can sprint on the treadmill for 20 seconds and then walk for 30 seconds).

The higher the intensity of each activity, typically the longer the rest/recovery time (e.g., If you sprint for 30 seconds you may need 45 seconds to 1 minute to recover by jogging or walking at a slower pace).

Interval Tip: Most cardio machines have programmed intervals. If you are not sure how to use your gym equipment, do not be afraid to ask for assistance.

Intensity Please!

In order to get the most bang for your buck, make sure you are putting in the right amount of INTENSITY into your intervals.

Intensity is the amount of effort you put into your exercise and one way to determine your effort is to use the R.P.E. (Rate of Perceived Exertion) scale.

What is the R.P.E. scale?

The R.P.E. is a subjective scale using the numbers zero through ten to rank your intensity (effort put into activity) during your physical activity.

By learning this scale, you can determine if you are putting enough effort into your interval sessions. This scale can be used for your resistance training routine as well.

R.P.E. SCALE	
0	NOTHING AT ALL
1	VERY LIGHT
2	FAIRLY LIGHT
3	MODERATE
4	SOMEWHAT HARD
5	HARD
6	
7	VERY HARD
8	
9	
10	VERY HARD (MAXIMAL Intensity)

Are You Tired of The Same Old Thing?

Doing cardio on a treadmill or elliptical can eventually become boring and cause overuse injuries due to performing the same movement patterns on a regular basis.

Besides, don't you get tired of the same old thing? Then, why not get creative with your cardio?

It's time to think outside the box and try the following cardio blast program.

This cardio blast routine will challenge your body by giving your mind a break from the monotony of your daily grind on the treadmill.

Items needed: Jump rope, bench or stable chair and medicine ball

Step 1: Gather needed items: Jump rope, bench or stable chair, medicine ball, your body.

Step 2: Identify your skill level (beginner, intermediate or advanced) and follow recommended sets and repetitions.

Step 3: Perform each exercise. At any point, adjust sets and repetitions according to your skill level and personal difficulty.

The following exercises are performed in a circuit fashion. Perform one exercise then move immediately to the next exercise without resting. Complete each exercise and then come to a state of rest.

General Warm-Up: Perform 5-10 minutes of light activity, such as jogging in place or walking on treadmill.

Jump Rope: Body standing straight with slight bend in knees. Hold rope lightly in hands. Turn rope, maintain soft bend in knees, stay on the base of feet. Do not pound feet on ground.

Step Ups: Stand in front of chair or bench with feet slightly apart and bend in knees. Keep upper body straight with core tight, arms by side. Slowly step up on bench with left foot, then right foot. Step back with opposite foot, until both feet are on ground, then repeat.

Med Ball Throw Downs: While standing straight, position med ball chest level using both hands. With a slight bend in knees, move body in an upward movement, bringing ball over head and then throwing ball toward ground. Let ball rebound, then catch. Repeat movement.

Line Hops: Create an imaginary line on the surface you are using. Stand behind imaginary line. While standing straight with slight bend in knees, jump forward over line, then jump back over same line in opposite direction. Keep a soft bend in knees throughout entire movement. Repeat.

Lateral Hops: Create an imaginary line on the surface you are using. Stand on the side of the imaginary line. While standing straight with slight bend in knees, jump over line in a lateral (side movement), then jump back over same line in opposite direction. Keep a soft bend in knees throughout entire movement. Repeat.

Beginners: Rest at least 1 min, 30 seconds after circuit is complete.

Sets	Performance Time	Repetitions
2-3	20-25 seconds	10-12

*Jump rope for 20-30 seconds

Intermediate: Rest 1 minute after entire circuit is complete.

Sets	Performance Time	Repetitions
3-4	25-40 seconds	15-20

* Jump rope for 30-45 seconds

Advanced: Rest 30-45 seconds after entire circuit is complete.

Sets	Performance Time	Repetitions
5-6	45 seconds – 1 minute	25-30

*Jump rope for 1 minute - 1 minute, 15 seconds

If or when you use cardio machines at the gym, please use the following guidelines to get the most out of your cardio sessions.

Cardio Guidelines

Do not lean on cardio machines: The handles that are provided on each cardio machine are not created for you to lean on. At all times keep body in an upright position with core tight. Leaning on the cardio machine takes away the effectiveness of the exercise by allowing the machines to support your body. Get the most out of every session and don't cheat yourself.

Pay Attention: If you are going to read while doing cardio, make sure your intensity level is sufficient enough to burn calories. Many people read and do not exert enough effort into their cardio. If you want to read, try using the recumbent bike where you can sit and read but still pedal fast.

Get Creative: Using the same cardio machines repeatedly can cause overuse injuries and mental burnout. It is good to mix up your cardio. If you like the bike, why not try adding the elliptical or the stair stepper?

Try Cardio Intervals: Why spend an hour walking slowly on the treadmill when you can spend 30-35 minutes doing intervals and burn more calories? Don't be afraid to try new things - it will shock your body and jump start your metabolism.

Chapter

A fit and flexible body is a healthier body!

18

Flexible and Fit

Stretching Essentials

There are numerous benefits to stretching, such as increased range of motion, decreased muscle stiffness and prevention of certain injuries. With so many benefits, stretching should be performed most days of the week following all physical activity. Choosing not to stretch on a regular basis can hinder your range of motion and lead to injuries.

Let's learn the basics of proper stretching.

What is range of motion (ROM)?

Range of motion is the pain free movement around a joint(s). The key word is pain free. As we age, we begin to experience stiffness of our joints and movements become painful as a result of not stretching on a regular basis. Chronic stiffness can lead to limited range of motion, which can lead to improper body mechanics and injuries.

Therefore, in order to avoid these issues, use the following guidelines to stretching and make stretching a regular part of your fitness training program.

Stretching Guidelines

Never stretch a cold muscle. Imagine placing a rubber band in the freezer for a period of time and then attempting to stretch it. It will not be as pliable cold as it would be at room temperature. Your muscles, ligaments and tendons are similar to a rubber band. The warmer they become, the more pliable they will be. This elasticity will help prevent injuries and increase your range of motion.

Stretch after your workout before complete cool down. Muscles need to have the ability to contract and produce force, therefore stretching too much before your workout could result in less force generated during your lifting.

Stretching is used to relax and elongate the muscles, and over stretching prior to resistance training may prevent optimal performance. In order to avoid this, stretch before you reach a cool down state immediately after your training session.

Never bounce. Your body has protective mechanisms which detect the length and force of a stretch. If you stretch your muscles too fast or too far, the body will respond by contracting the muscles. Do not force your body to go beyond its normal range of motion by bouncing or forcing yourself into a stretched position. Forcing your body to go beyond this point can lead to injuries.

Stretch at least three days per week. Regular stretching will provide a greater range of motion to perform Activities of Daily Living (ADLs) such as grocery shopping, gardening and cleaning. Being flexible will, in addition, help you with sports-related performances and lessen chances of injury.

Follow the F.I.T.T. Model for Stretching

The F.I.T.T. model below teaches you the frequency, intensity, type and time for stretching.

Frequency: At least three days per week, preferably daily and after all physical activity

Intensity: Slow, controlled and not forced. Slowly elongate muscle with low level of force

Type: At least 4-5 stretches per major muscle groups (legs, arms, chest, back)

Time: 15- 30 second holds (static stretching)

The following stretches can be performed after each workout. Remember each stretching guideline and do not force your body beyond its normal range of motion.

Upper Body Stretches
(Shoulders, Back, Triceps, Chest, Biceps)

Triceps Stretch (standing)

Stand in an upright position with a slight bend in knees. Raise your arm over your head and bend your elbow all the way so your hand is behind your neck. Use your opposite arm to stabilize your elbow. Hold for 15-30 seconds. Repeat 3 to 5 times and then perform stretch on the opposite side.

Triceps Stretch (sitting)

Sit in a chair with body in an upright position, core tight and shoulders back. Raise your arm over your head and bend your elbow all the way so your hand is behind your neck. Use your opposite arm to stabilize your elbow. Hold for 15-30 seconds. Repeat 3 to 5 times and then perform stretch on the opposite side.

Shoulder Rolls

Begin sitting or standing with your arms at your sides. Shrug your shoulders up. While your shoulders are in the shrugged position, slowly roll them forward and down. Repeat this movement 5 to 10 times. Then do shoulder shrugs and rolls backward, and repeat this movement 5 to 10 times.

Biceps Stretch

Take your arms out to the sides, slightly behind your elbows, with the thumbs up. Rotate your thumbs down and back until they are pointing to the back wall. You will feel a stretch in your biceps. Repeat 3 to 5 times.

Reaching Up and Down

While sitting or standing with your arms at your sides, reach up with one hand toward the ceiling and reach down with the other hand toward the floor. Hold this stretch for 15 to 30 seconds. Repeat 3 to 5 times while alternating arms.

Anterior Shoulder Stretch

Stand in a doorway or use a sturdy object (tree, pole) with your right arm out to your side at a 90-degree angle and your elbow flexed to 90 degrees. Place your palm, forearm, and elbow on the door frame (tree/pole). Lean forward through the open door, feeling the stretch in your anterior chest and shoulder. Hold this position for 15 to 30 seconds. Repeat 3 to 5 times and then perform stretch on the opposite side.

Upper Back Stretch

Stand in an upright position, feet together with slight bend in knees. Next, clasps hands in front of body and round back towards floor, pressing arms away from body. You will feel a stretch in the upper part of your back. Keep head in a neutral (head aligned straight) position throughout movement. Hold position. Repeat 3 to 5 times.

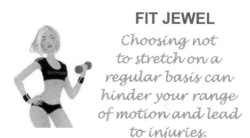

FIT JEWEL

Choosing not to stretch on a regular basis can hinder your range of motion and lead to injuries.

Lower Body Stretches
(Glutes, Hamstrings and Calves)

Gluteal (buttocks) Stretch

Sit in a chair or lie on your back. Flex (bend) one knee toward your chest and place your hands around the front of your knee, pulling the knee up towards the shoulder of the same side and you will feel the stretch in your gluteal (buttocks) area. Hold position for 15 to 30 seconds. Repeat 3 to 5 times and then perform stretch on the opposite side.

Hip Flexor (hips) Stretch

Stand with your hands grasping a chair or sturdy object (tree). With your left foot supporting your body weight and right leg extended back, push your pelvis forward with your torso in the upright position, you will feel the stretch in the front of your hip. Hold this position for 15 to 30 seconds. Repeat 3 to 5 times and then perform stretch on the opposite side.

Hamstring Stretch (Standing)

While standing, place one foot forward on a bench or step with knee slightly bent. While supporting most of your weight on the other foot, lean forward at the waist with arms reaching toward your toes, you will feel the stretch in the back of your thigh (hamstrings). Hold this position for 15 to 30 seconds. Repeat 3 to 5 times and then perform stretch on the opposite side.

Hamstring Stretch (Lying Down)

Lie on your back, place one leg in the air, while opposite leg rests on the floor. With slight bend in knee, position hands underneath your knee and gently move knee towards chest, you will feel the stretch in your hamstring. Hold this position for 15 to 30 seconds. Repeat 3 to 5 times and then perform stretch on the opposite side.

Quadriceps (front part of leg) Stretch

Standing with your right hand grasping a chair for stability, hold your left ankle behind you with your left hand, pulling it upward and backward and feeling the stretch in the front of your thigh. Hold this position for 15 to 30 seconds. Repeat 3 to 5 times and then perform stretch on the opposite side.

Calf Stretch (Bent Knee)

Standing with your arms stretched in front of you and hands on a wall, support your weight on the right foot with the right knee slightly bent while placing your left foot behind you with the heel on the ground and the knee slightly bent. Lean forward, you will feel the stretch in your calf. Hold for 15 to 30 seconds. Repeat 3 to 5 times. Perform this stretch on the opposite side.

Calf Stretch (Straight Knee)

Standing with your arms stretched in front of you and hands on a wall, support your weight on your right foot with knee slightly bent while placing your left foot behind you with the heel on the ground and the knee straight. Lean forward, you will feel the stretch in your calf. Hold for 15 to 30 seconds. Repeat 3 to 5 times. Perform this stretch on the opposite side.

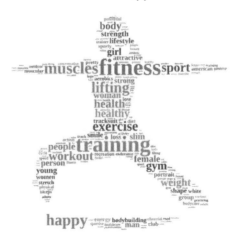

Chapter

It's your body and your curves, embrace yourself!

19

Define Your Curves

Let The Toning Begin

If you're a beginning Fitness Queen, it is essential to slowly incorporate resistance training into your fitness training program at least 3 days per week on non-consecutive days (Monday, Wednesday and Friday). Doing more than 3 days per week at the beginning of your fitness training program may result in mental burn out and injuries. In addition to performing resistance training as a part of your new fitness training program, it is also recommended to incorporate cardiovascular exercise on the same day as your resistance training. On the days in which you choose to perform both resistance training and cardiovascular activities, perform your resistance training exercises first followed by your cardiovascular activities. Following this pattern of movement has been shown to be beneficial due to the different energy systems the body utilizes during resistance training and cardiovascular activities.

Intermediate and advanced Fitness Queens, you can incorporate resistance training 5 days per week into your fitness training program. At this stage you have the strength to perform more volume. In addition to your resistance training, perform cardiovascular activities 5 days a week, allowing at least 48 hours of rest in between each muscle group. The body's muscle fibers are broken down when you resistance train, therefore rest time is essential in assisting your body in recovery and repair.

Before you begin the following exercises to sculpt your curves, identify your current fitness training level. Identifying your current fitness training level will assist you in choosing the proper amount of sets, repetitions and rest time for each exercise.

Identify Your Fitness Training Level

Identify whether or not you're beginner, intermediate or advanced level. Based on your training level, determine how many sets and repetitions you will perform for each exercise.

Below is a description of each training level.

> **Beginner:** No previous experience with resistance training or recreational activities.

> **Intermediate:** Train at least 3 days per week, including cardiovascular activities.

> **Advanced:** An athlete or you have more than a year experience with resistance training. Train at least 4-5 days per week.

Sets and Repetitions

Below you find the amount of sets and repetitions that you will perform based on your current fitness level.

> **Beginner:** Perform: 2 sets per exercise for 10-12 repetitions using light weight (5-8 lbs). Perform modified version (MV) for each exercise that isn't within your current fitness level.

> **Intermediate:** Perform: 3 sets per exercise for 12-15 repetitions each using moderate weight (10-15 lbs).

> **Advanced:** Perform 3-5 sets per exercise for 6-8 repetitions for strength and 12-15 repetitions for tone. Use moderate to heavier weight (15 lbs or more).

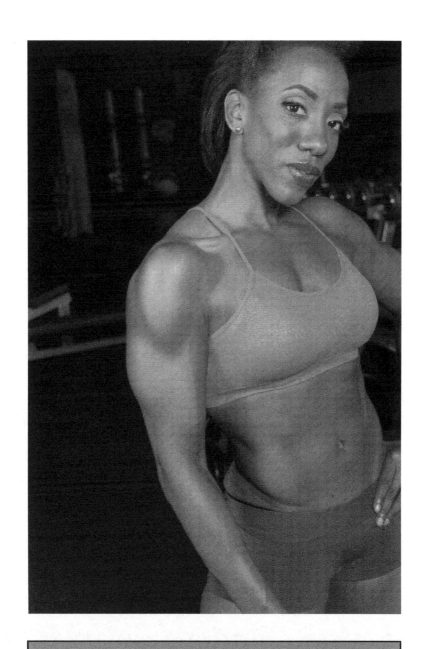

Upper Body Exercises

Tighten, Firm and Tone

A strong and toned upper body not only looks great for the warmer months when sleeveless shirts and swimsuits are worn, but toned arms are also great for assisting you in activities of daily living such as picking up your children, carrying groceries and being able lift and carry your laundry. Research has shown that after the age of 30 women begin to lose muscle tissue by 3 to 5 percent per decade. A loss of muscle tissue can lead to diminished mobility and strength in the aging process; therefore, it is essential to incorporate resistance training into your normal fitness regimen on a regular basis.

The following exercises in this chapter will help you sculpt and tone your upper body without adding a bulky appearance. Discover your skill level and perform the exercises prescribed to you. If you are a beginner, listen to your body and only perform the amount of sets and repetitions that feel appropriate for you. Intermediate and advanced levels - don't be afraid to safely push your body by adding extra resistance and increasing your repetitions.

Chest Exercises

Movement Tip: To avoid injury, keep core contracted throughout entire movement. Doing so will keep body aligned and lessen the chance of injury to your back.

Beginner Level

Exercise	Sets	Repetitions
One-Arm Med Ball Pushups *Modified Version	2-3	4-6
Single-Legged Chest Press	2-3	8-10 each arm
Physio-ball Chest Press	2-3	10-12 each arm
Resistance Band Flyes	2-3	10-12

Intermediate Level

Exercise	Sets	Repetitions
One-Arm Med Ball Pushups	3-4	15-20
Single-Legged Chest Press	3-4	15-20 each arm
Physio-ball Chest Press	3-4	15-20 each arm
Physio-ball Pushups	3-4	10-15
Resistance Band Flyes	3-4	12-15

Advanced Level

Exercise	Sets	Repetitions
One-Arm Med Ball Pushups	4-5	15
Single-Legged Chest Press	4-5	15
Physio-ball Chest Press	4-5	15 each arm
One-Arm Med Ball Pushups	4-5	15
Resistance Band Flyes	4-5	15-20

One-Arm Med Ball Pushups

Targeted Muscles: chest, triceps

Set Up: Kneel on the ground with hands positioned shoulder width apart, one hand resting on med ball with other hand placed on ground. From kneeling position, extend arms and legs.

Action: In a slow and controlled manner, bend your elbows and lower your body until arms form a 90-degree angle. Hold for a count and then extend your arms and push body back to starting position. Complete set and then switch arms.

Movement Tip: To avoid back injury, keep core tight and body in straight position. Do not drop hips.

*Modified Version: Perform exercise on your knees.

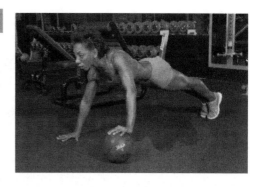

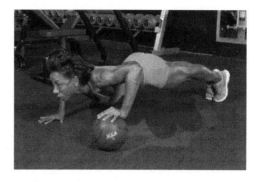

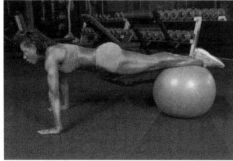

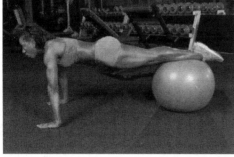

Physio-ball Pushups

Targeted Muscles: chest, triceps

Set Up: Place stability ball in front of body. Slowly roll your body onto the ball until your shins rest on ball. Your arms are positioned shoulder width apart with lower body and core tight. Keep slight bend in elbows.

Action: In a slow and controlled manner, bend elbows and slowly lower body until your arms form a 90- degree angle. Hold for a count and then extend arms to return body to starting position. Repeat movement until set is complete.

Movement Tip: To avoid injury, keep core tight throughout entire movement.

Single-Legged Chest Press

Targeted Muscles: glutes, hamstrings, chest, triceps

Set Up: Lay on back with both feet on ground, knees bent with arms bent holding dumbbells at chest level.

Action: In an upward movement, slowly bridge up on one leg, with opposite leg elevated off ground. Once lower body is off ground, press dumbbell upward until arms are fully extended. Hold for a count and then bring body back to starting position. Complete set and then switch to opposite arm and leg.

*Modified Version: Keep both feet on ground. Maintain body in bridged position.

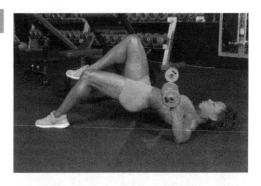

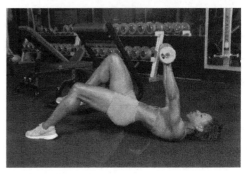

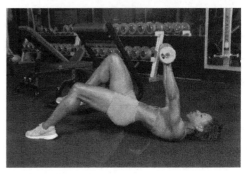

Physio-ball Chest Press

Targeted Muscles: chest, triceps

Set Up: Position body on a stability ball with a pair of dumbbells in both hands with feet positioned apart. In a slow and controlled manner, slowly walk your feet away from the ball until your upper back rests on stability ball. Elbows are bent with dumbbells facing inward with hips parallel to floor and feet positioned slightly apart.

Action: In a slow and controlled manner, slowly lower weight to sides of upper chest until slight stretch is felt in chest or shoulder. Hold for a count and then slowly extend arms to starting position without locking elbows. Keep core engaged and hips elevated in order to maintain form throughout entire movement.

Movement Tip: Keep hips and core contracted.

*Modified Version: Drop hips to mid-level. Keep core contracted at all times.

Chest Press with Bridge

Targeted Muscles: glutes, hamstring and chest

Set Up: Lay on your back with knees bent, feet flat on floor, elbows bent while holding medicine ball at chest level.

Action: In a slow and controlled manner, lift body off mat by squeezing glutes and hamstrings in an upward movement (bridge), while keeping ball near chest. Once hips are off ground, extend arms and press ball towards ceiling. When balls returns, catch ball with slight bend in elbows. Bring lower body down from bridge movement and repeat entire movement.

Movement Tip: Find a focal point on the ceiling when tossing the ball. This will allow to you to remain consistent with pressing the ball upward and catching it in the same spot.

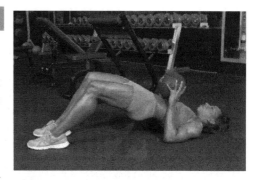

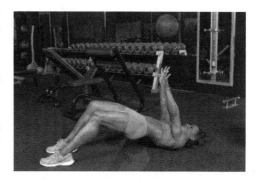

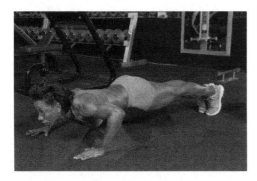

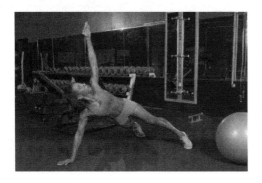

Around the World

Targeted Muscles: chest, triceps

Set Up: Begin in pushup position with hands shoulder width apart, body in a straight line, core and lower body tight.

Action: In a slow and controlled manner, slowly bend your elbows and lower body until you reach a 90-degree angle. Hold for a count and then extend your arms and return to starting position. While in starting pushup position, lift right arm and rotate arm across body and hold for a count. Bring arm down. Perform another pushup and then repeat lift with opposite arm.

*Modified Version: Perform exercise on knees.

Targeted Muscles: chest, triceps

Set Up: While in a standing position, with chest up shoulder blades back and slight bend in knees, grab resistant band and place behind the back of your shoulders. Once band is placed behind shoulders place a bend in elbows with arms extended out to the side of your body.

Action: With a slight bend in elbows, squeeze chest muscles together and bring arms together with palms facing one another. Hold for account and bring arms back to starting position. Repeat until set is complete.

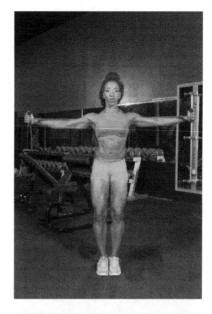

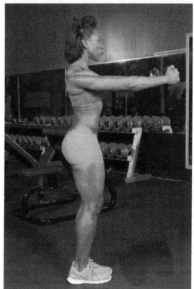

FIT JEWEL

Using resistance training bands is a non-expensive and fun way to get fit at the gym, at home or while you travel. If you travel often, packing a resistance training band in your suitcase will allow you to stay fit on the go. You can get fit and creative with resistance training bands!

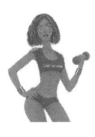

Movement Tip: Keep core contracted while performing each exercise. This will keep body aligned and lessen the chance of injury to your back.

Beginner Level

Exercise	Sets	Repetitions
Seated Resistance Band Rows	2-3	10-12
One-Arm Row	2-3	10-12
Two-Arm Row *Modified Version	2-3	10-12

Intermediate Level

Exercise	Sets	Repetitions
Seated Resistance Band Rows	3-4	15-20
One-Arm Row	3-4	15-20
Two-Arm Row	3-4	15-20

Advanced Level

Exercise	Sets	Repetitions
Seated Resistance Band Rows	4-5	8-15
One-Arm Row	4-5	8-15
Two-Arm Row	4-5	15

Seated Resistance Band Rows

Targeted Muscles: back, chest

Set Up: While in a seated position, shoulder back, core engaged and chest up, with knees bent and heels on the ground, place resistance band under the base of your shoe, grasping both handles with arms fully extended.

Action: In a slow and controlled manner, bring elbows back by squeezing shoulder blades together. Hold for a count and repeat entire movement until set is complete.

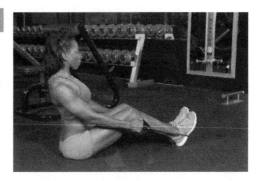

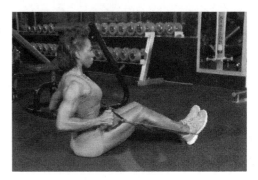

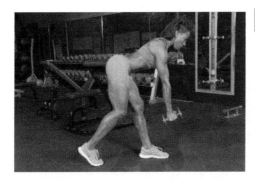

One-Arm Row

Targeted Muscles: back, core

Set Up: Begin by standing in a split stance, with one foot staggered in front of the other. Place a slight bend in knees, arm holding dumbbells in front of body with slight lean in torso.

Action: In a slow and controlled manner with core engaged, bring elbow back by squeezing your shoulder blade. Hold for a count and then extend arm back to starting position. Complete movement until set is complete and then switch arms.

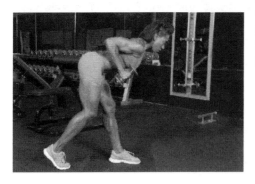

Two-Arm Row

Targeted Muscles: back, core

Set Up: Begin by standing in a split stance, with one foot staggered in front of the other. Place a slight bend in knees, lean in torso, with arms extended in front of body holding dumbbells.

Action: In a slow and controlled manner with core engaged, bring elbows back by squeezing your shoulder blades together. Hold for a count and then extend arms back to starting position. Complete movement until set is complete.

*Modified Version: Keep torso forward, but keep back leg on the ground.

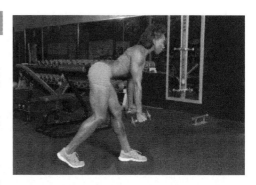

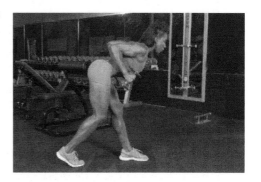

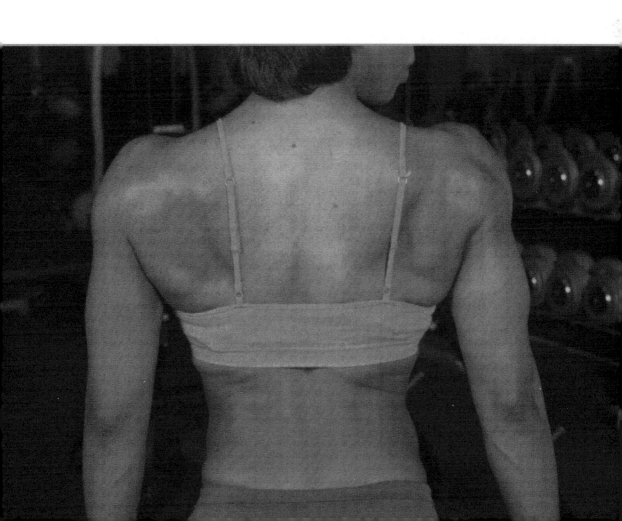

Shoulder Exercises

Movement Tip: Keep core contracted while performing each exercise. This will keep body aligned and lessen the chance of injury to your back.

Beginner Level

Exercise	Sets	Repetitions
Core Shoulder Lifts *Modified Version	2-3	8-10
Front Shoulder Raises	2-3	10-12
Lateral Shoulder Raises	2-3	10-12
Rear Shoulder Raises	2-3	10-12

Intermediate Level

Exercise	Sets	Repetitions
Core Shoulder Lifts	3-4	10-12
Front Shoulder Raises	3-4	15-20
Lateral Shoulder Raises	3-4	15-20
Rear Shoulder Raises	3-4	15-20

Advanced Level

Exercise	Sets	Repetitions
Core Shoulder Lifts*	4	12-15
Front Shoulder Raises	4-5	8-15
Lateral Shoulder Raises	4-5	8-15
Rear Shoulder Raises	4-5	8-15

*Use a heavier medicine ball around 8-10 lbs. for added resistance

Core Shoulder Lifts

Targeted Muscles: anterior deltoids (front shoulder), core

Set Up: Position body on a mat with feet flat on floor, knees bent, chest up and arms extended in front of body while holding medicine ball.

Action: With core tight, in a slow and controlled manner, slightly lean back and raise feet about 2 inches off ground (Advanced level can raise feet higher). Once stabilized in position, lift arms in an upward position. Hold for a count, and then bring arms down. Repeat movement.

Movement Tip: Keep core tight and chest up to avoid rounding back while performing movement.

***Modified Version:** Keep both feet on ground.

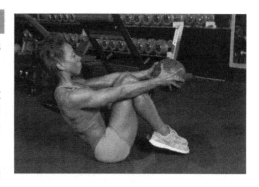

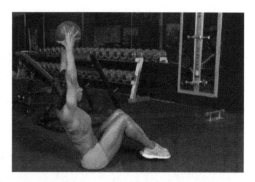

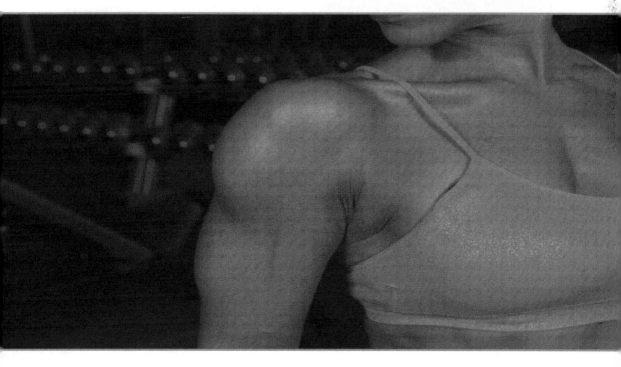

Front Shoulder Raises

Targeted Muscles: anterior deltoids (front shoulder)

Set up: Stand in an upright position, feet positioned together or apart, core engaged with slight bend in knees. Dumbbells held in a neutral (palms facing inward towards your body) position in your hands.

Action: In a slow and controlled manner lift dumbbells in an upward movement raising arms until they reach eye level with palms facing each other. Hold for a count and then return hands back to starting position.

Movement tip: Keep slight bend in knees throughout the entire movement and don't allow body to swing as you move the dumbbells away from your body. Keep core engaged and feet anchored to ground in order to avoid swinging movement.

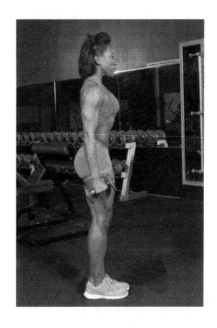

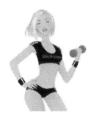

FIT JEWEL

Hello summer and short sleeve shirts!

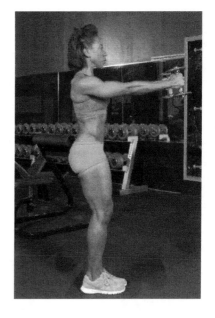

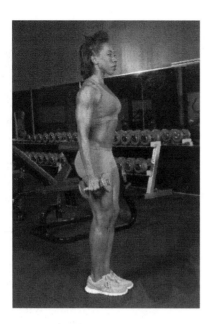

Lateral Shoulder Raises

Targeted Muscles: lateral deltoids (middle of shoulder)

Set Up: Stand with your feet together, knees slightly bent, while holding dumbbells facing inward towards your hips.

Action: With a slight bend in elbows, in a slow and controlled manner, lift arms in a lateral position (lateral means away from the mid-line of your body) until arms are parallel to the floor. Hold for a count and then lower arms back to starting position. Repeat movement until set is complete.

Movement Tip: Do not bring arms too high. As a reference point, you should be able to see the back of your hands in your peripheral view. If you can't see your hands, you're lifting too high. Raising arms to high releases tension off shoulder and places stress on other muscles. Do not arch back throughout movement.

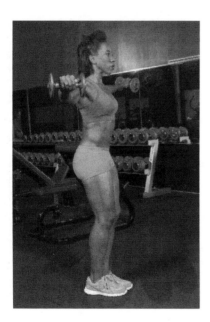

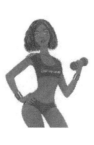

FIT JEWEL

Toned shoulders look great regardless of what you wear, therefore don't forget to incorporate shoulder exercises into your fitness training program.

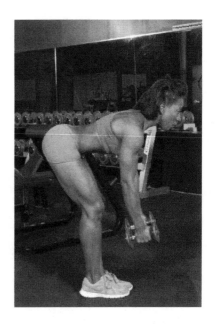

Targeted Muscles: rear deltoids, core

Set Up: Begin with feet together, knees bent, torso forward with arms extended in front of body holding dumbbells facing inward towards body.

Action: With a slight bend in elbows, in a slow and controlled manner, lift arms away from body in an arching movement by squeezing shoulder blades together. Hold for a count and then lower arms back to starting position. Repeat movement until set is complete.

Movement Tip: Keep knees bent and core tight.

FIT JEWEL

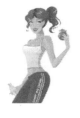

Nice toned shoulders are great for the winter, summer or anytime of the year!

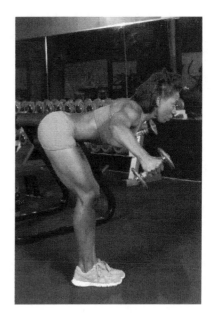

Movement Tip: Keep core contracted while performing each exercise. This will keep body aligned and lessen the chance of injury to your back.

Beginner Level

Exercise	Sets	Repetitions
Kneeling Physio-ball Curls	2-3	8-10
Single-Legged Bicep Curls *Modified Version	2-3	8-10
Split Stance Hammer Curls	2-3	8-10
Resistance Bands Curls	2-3	8-10

Intermediate Level

Exercise	Sets	Repetitions
Kneeling Physio-ball Curls	3-4	10-12
Single-Legged Bicep Curls	3-4	10-12
Split Stance Bicep Curls	3-4	10-12
Resistance Bands Curls	3-4	10-12

Advanced Level

Exercise	Sets	Repetitions
Kneeling Physio-ball Curls	4-5	12-15
Single-Legged Bicep Curls	4-5	12-15
Split Stance Bicep Curls	4-5	12-15
Resistance Bands Curls	4-5	12-15

Targeted Muscles: biceps

Set Up: Kneel down in front of physio-ball with elbows positioned on ball, with palms facing upward while holding dumbbells along with core engaged.

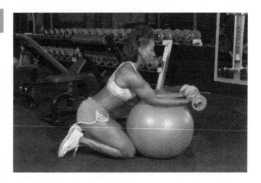

Action: In a slow and controlled manner, squeeze biceps and bring down dumbbells towards your shoulders, keeping elbows close to body. Hold for a count and then extend arms without full extension of elbow back to starting position. Repeat movement until set is complete.

Movement Tip: Keep core tight to avoid hurting your lower back and if you experience knee problems, place a mat or towel under knees.

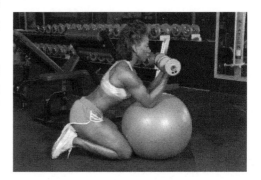

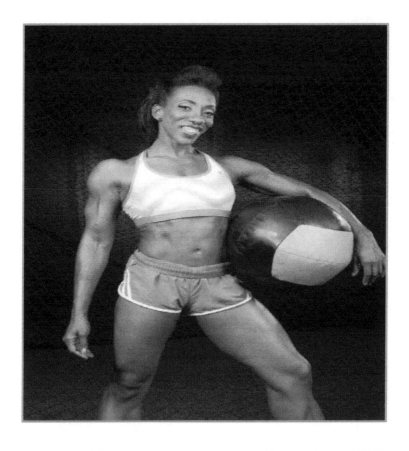

Targeted Muscles: biceps, core

Set Up: Stand with both feet together, slight bend in knees. Arms positioned by side, with palms facing away from your body while holding dumbbells.

Action: In a slow and controlled manner, slowly lift one leg off ground. Once stabilized, with elbow locked near side, curl dumbbell upward by squeezing biceps. Hold for a count and then lower arms back to starting position without locking out elbows. Repeat movement until set is complete and then switch leg to balance on.

Movement Tip: Slowly bring arms down without fully extending them.

*Modified Version: Keep both feet on ground or bring foot slightly off the ground.

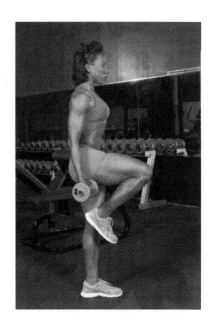

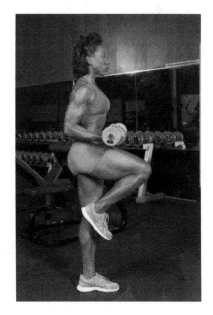

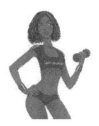

FIT JEWEL

While standing on one leg, keep core engaged this will help you keep your balance.

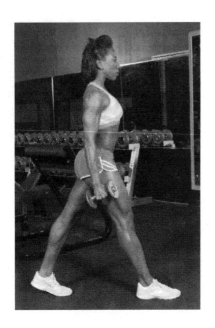

Split Stance Hammer Curls

Targeted Muscles: biceps

Set Up: In an upright position stagger feet evenly positioning body weight on front and back legs, with shoulders back, core engaged while holding dumbbells in a neutral position (palms facing towards your body), with slight bend in elbows.

Action: In a slow and controlled manner, slowly squeeze biceps and bring dumbbells towards your shoulder while keeping elbows positioned close to your body. Hold for a count and then return hands to starting position without fully extending arms. Repeat movement until set is complete.

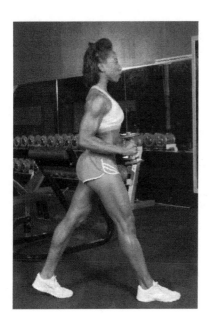

FIT JEWEL

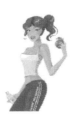

Never jeopardize form for weight. If you can't properly lift the weight you're using, decrease the amount of weight.

Targeted Muscles: biceps

Set Up: Place resistance band underneath both feet creating enough space to create equal resistance on handles. Once band is placed under feet, stand in an upright position with shoulders back, core engaged, slight bend in knees and palms facing upward with resistance band in both hands.

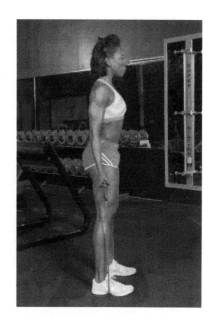

Action: In a slow and controlled manner with elbows close to body, squeeze biceps and bring hands towards shoulders, hold for a count and then return hands to starting position without fully extending arms.

Movement Tip: Keep a slight bend in knees at all times in order to avoid placing stress on your lower back. When performing movement, do not allow elbows to move away from the body, doing so will place less stress on biceps.

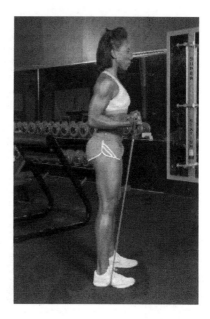

FIT JEWEL

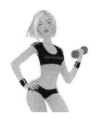

Keep elbows locked into your side in order to fully make the biceps work.

Tricep Exercises

Movement Tip: Keep core contracted while performing each exercise. This will keep body aligned and lessen the chance of injury to your back.

Beginner Level

Exercise	Sets	Repetitions
Resistance Band Extensions	1-2	8-10
Standing Triceps Kickbacks	1-2	8-10
Seated Overhead Triceps Extensions *Modified Version	1-2	8-10

Intermediate Level

Exercise	Sets	Repetitions
Resistance Band Extensions	2-3	10-12
Standing Triceps Kickbacks	2-3	10-12
Seated Overhead Triceps Extensions	2-3	10-12
Pyramid Pushups	2-3	10-12

Advanced Level

Exercise	Sets	Repetitions
Resistance Band Extensions	3-4	12-15
Standing Triceps Kickbacks	3-4	12-15
Seated Overhead Triceps Extensions	3-4	12-15
Physio-ball Triceps Pushups	3-4	12-15

Resistance Band Extensions

Targeted Muscles: Triceps

Set Up: Place resistance band underneath the back of your foot and then stand in an upright position staggering feet evenly in order to position body weight on front and back legs. Shoulders back, core engaged while holding resistance band in hand with elbow bent.

Action: In a slow and controlled manner, contract core and fully extend arm by squeezing triceps without locking out your elbow. Hold for a count and then return arm back to starting position. Repeat movement until set is complete and then switch your arm and foot.

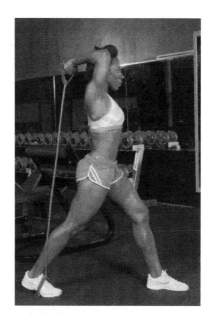

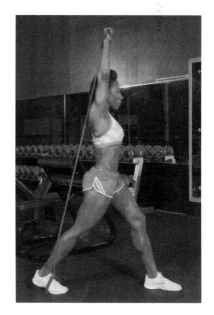

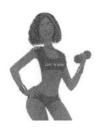

FIT JEWEL

Performing these exercises will give you the confidence to wave goodbye!

One-Arm Triceps Extensions

Targeted Muscles: triceps, core

Set Up: Place body in push up position, with hands positioned shoulder width apart. Legs spread apart to form a V with dumbbells in front of body.

Action: While contracting core, slowly grab dumbbell off floor and lift right arm off ground, tucking right elbow at side. Once elbow is tucked into side, in a slow and controlled manner, extend arm without locking out. Repeat movement until set is complete and then switch arms. Complete set with opposite arm.

Movement Tip: To avoid back injuries, keep core contracted throughout entire movement.

*Modified version: Perform on knees.

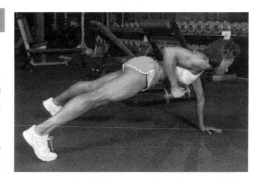

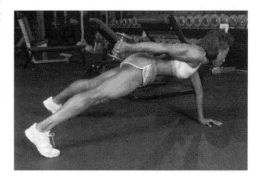

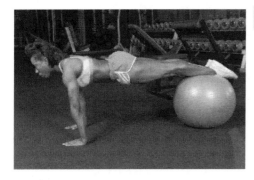

Physio-ball Triceps Pushups

Targeted Muscles: triceps, core

Set Up: In a slow and controlled manner, roll body forward onto stability ball until shins are resting on ball. Hands are positioned closer than shoulder width, with slight bend in elbows.

Action: In a slow and controlled manner, bend elbows in a hinge movement and lower body about 2-4 inches from the ground. Hold for a count and then extend arms to return body to starting position. Repeat movement until set is complete.

Movement Tip: To help balance on ball, keep core contracted and lower body aligned.

*Modified Version: Do not use ball, instead use mat and perform exercise on knees. Keep core tight throughout entire movement.

Standing Triceps Kickbacks

Targeted Muscles: triceps, core

Set Up: Stand with feet together, slight bend in knees. Torso forward and elbows tucked into side of body while holding dumbbells in a supinated position (hands facing upwards towards your body).

Action: In a slow and controlled manner, extend your arms by squeezing your triceps. Hold for a count and then bring arms back to starting position. Repeat movement until set is complete.

Movement Tip: Fully extend arms without locking elbows.

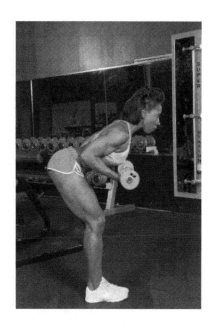

FIT JEWEL

To avoid overuse injuries at the elbow joint, don't lock out elbows on triceps exercises.

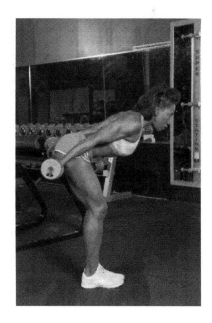

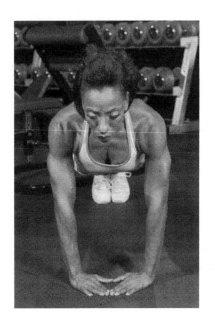

Targeted Muscles: triceps, core and chest

Set Up: Start with body in a pushup position, hands are positioned close together with index fingers and thumbs touching to form a diamond. Lower body and core remain aligned and contracted.

Action: In a slow and controlled manner, bend elbows and lower body parallel to floor. Once arms are positioned at 90-degrees, stop movement. Hold for a count and then extend arms to return to starting position. Repeat movement until set is complete. Do not lockout elbows when returning to starting position.

Movement Tip: To avoid back injuries, keep core tight throughout entire movement.

*Modified Version: Perform exercise on knees.

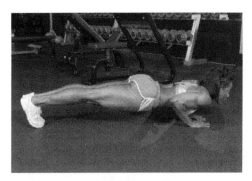

FIT JEWEL

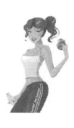

Many women have weaker upper bodies, but performing this exercise will help improve your upper body strength and tone your arms.

Seated Overhead Triceps Extensions

Targeted Muscles: triceps, core

Set Up: Place body on a stability ball while holding dumbbells. In a slow and controlled manner, walk your feet away from ball until your upper back rests on stability ball. Hips parallel to the floor with arms extended holding dumbbells.

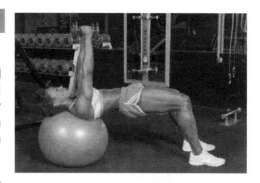

Action: While maintaining balance on stability ball, in a slow and controlled manner, bend elbows and lower weight until your elbows are fully bent. Hold for a count and then extend arms back to starting position. Repeat movement until set is complete.

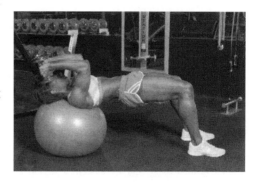

*Movement Tip: Extend arms without locking elbows.

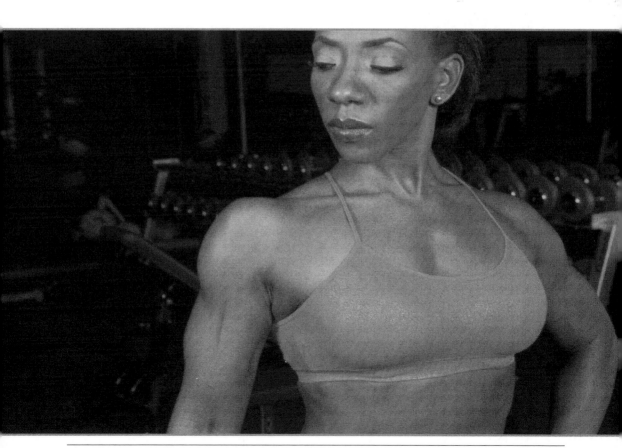

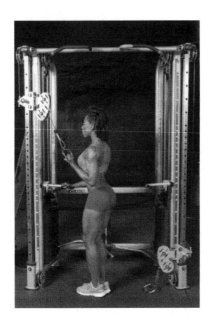

Targeted Muscles: triceps, core

Set up: Stand in an upright position with body facing towards triceps extension attachment either on a Smith Machine or Universal Cable System. Shoulder blades back, slight bend in knees, core engaged and hand positioned in supinated position (palms facing upward).

Action: In a slow and controlled manner fully extend arm by squeezing tricep. Extend arm without locking elbow. Hold for a count and then return arm back to starting position. Repeat movement until set is complete and then switch arms.

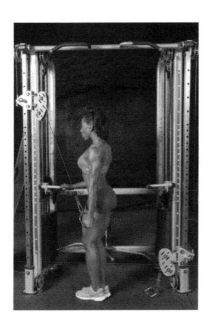

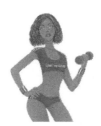

FIT JEWEL

Using the cable machine is a great way to add variety into your resistance training program.

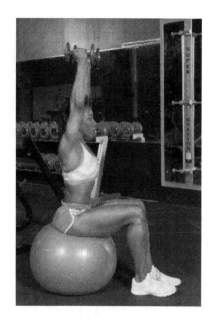

Targeted Muscles: triceps, core

Set Up: Sit on physio-ball with slight bend in knees, feet flat on ground, core engaged, shoulders back and arms extended holding dumbbells.

Action: While maintaining stability on ball, in a slow and controlled manner, bend elbows and lower weight until your hands are behind your head. Hold for a count and then extend arms back to starting position. Repeat movement until set is complete.

Movement Tip: Extend arms without locking elbows out.

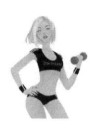

FIT JEWEL

Performing exercises on an unstable object such as the physio-ball is a great way to build core strength and balance.

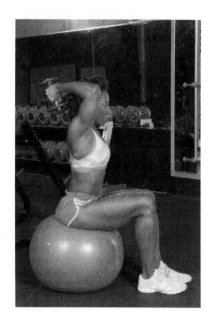

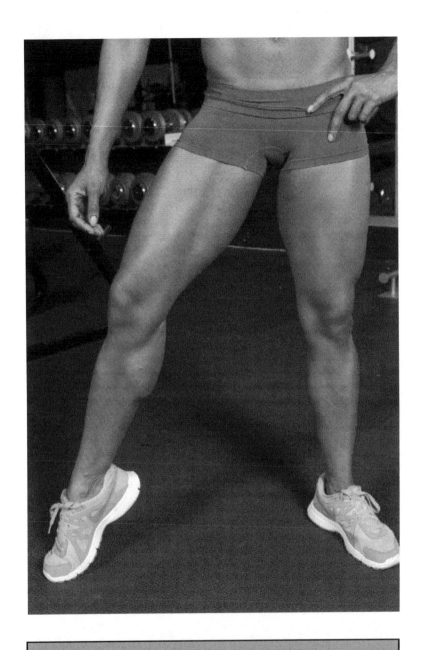

Lower Body Exercises

Hips, Glutes and Thighs, Oh My!

Have you ever turned around and looked at your backside and thought, "I wish my backside was firmer?" Whether you are 26 or 46, at some point in time most women have made this statement to themselves. The backside, or the glutes and the thighs, for many women are the hardest and most challenging area to firm, tighten and tone. Women naturally carry more body fat in these areas, and as a result find it harder to see the tone they desire. Do you find it hard to tone these areas of your body?

If this is you, the exercises on the following pages are designed not only to help you look great in your favorite jeans, but the following exercises are also designed to help you keep your legs strong enough to run, bike, dance and perform all other activities of living. A firmer backside and toned legs are only a few squats away, what are you waiting for?

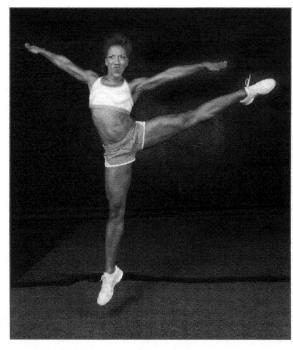

Firm, tightened and toned legs not only look great in a pair of jeans or shorts, they are also great for jumping and other sporting activities

Lower Body Exercises

Movement Tip: Keep core contracted while performing each exercise. This will keep body aligned and lessen the chance of injury to your back.

Exercise Tip: In order to make lunges and squats more difficult, add dumbbells.

Beginner Level

Exercise	Sets	Repetitions
Reverse Lunges	1-2	10-12
Hamstring Blast	1-2	10-12
Hamstring Reach	1-2	10-12
Frog Lifts	1-2	10-12

Intermediate Level

Exercise	Sets	Repetitions
Squat Kicks	2-3	12-15
Lunge Ups	2-3	12-15
Single Legged Bridges	2-3	12-15
Frog Lifts	2-3	12-15

Advanced Level

Exercise	Sets	Repetitions
Squat Kicks	3-4	15-20
Frog Lifts	3-4	15-20
Single Legged Bridges	3-4	15-20
Hamstring Reaches	3-4	15-20
Lateral Lunges	3-4	15-20

Reverse Lunges

Targeted Muscles: quadriceps, glutes and hamstrings

Set Up: Stand with feet together, slight bend in knees with hands resting on hips or placed in front of body.

Action: With chest up and core tight, in a slow and controlled manner, step back with one leg, creating a wide stance between your front and back leg. Keep a slight bend in both knees without knees going over toes. Your back knee approaches the ground but never touches the ground. Hold for a count and push off back leg, bring back leg forward to starting position. Repeat movement until set is complete on one leg and then switch legs and repeat movement.

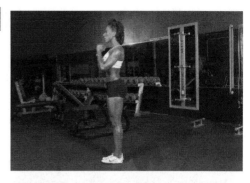

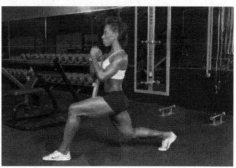

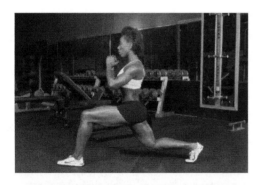

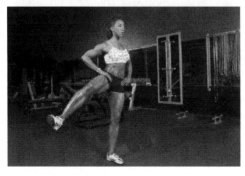

Reverse Lunge with Abductions

Targeted Muscles: quadriceps, glutes and hamstrings

Set Up: Stand with feet together, slight bend in knees, shoulders back, core engaged with hands resting on hips.

Action: In a slow and controlled manner, step back with one leg, creating a wide stance between your front and back leg. Keep a slight bend in both knees without knees going over toes. Your back knee approaches the ground but never touches the ground. Once in this position, hold for a count and then bring back leg forward to starting position.

From starting position, place sight bend in lead leg and move your leg away from the midline (middle) of your body. Hold for a count and then bring leg back to starting position. Switch legs and repeat movements with opposite leg.

Squat with Side Kick

Targeted Muscles: Glutes, hamstrings

Set Up: Stand with feet hip width apart, core tight and shoulder blades retracted

Action: In a slow and controlled manner, engage core and squat until your knees make a 90 degree angle. Hold squat for a count while maintaining proper form. Return completely from squat, shift weight onto right leg, and then kick out to the left side of your body. Bring leg back to ground, repeat squatting movement and perform kick with opposite leg.

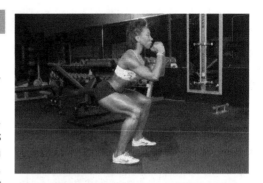

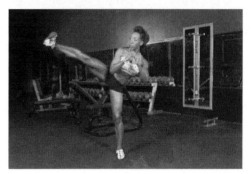

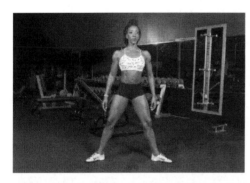

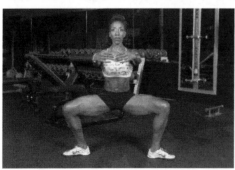

Plie Squats with Calf Raises

Targeted Muscles: calves, inner thighs, glutes

Set Up: Stand with feet wider than shoulder width apart, toes turned outward with core engaged and arms extended by body.

Action: In a slow and controlled manner, lower body until your thighs are parallel to the ground. Keep knees pointed in same direction as toes. Hold for a count and then return body back to starting position. While in an upward position, lift up on calves and perform a calve raise. Bring calves down. Repeat entire movement until set is complete.

*Movement Tip: Keep core contracted throughout entire movement. Do not allow knees to go over toes.

Lateral Lunges

Targeted Muscles: Glutes, hamstrings

Set Up: Place feet together or hip-width apart with your toes pointed directly forward. Shoulders back, core engaged and hands placed in front of body or positioned on hips.

Action: In a slow and controlled manner, lift your right leg and step to the side. Once your foot is fully planted, push your hips back and bend your right knee to lower into a lunge. Descend until your right thigh is about parallel to the floor and then extend your hips and knee to come back up.

Return your right foot to the starting position and then perform the next repetition, stepping to the side with your left foot. Continue this back and forth movement pattern until you complete set.

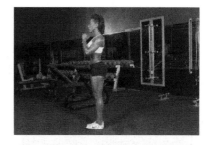
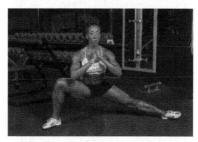
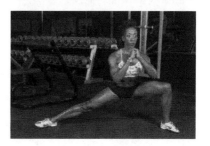

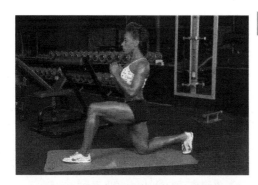
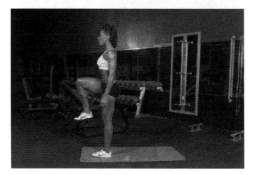

Lunge Ups

Targeted Muscles: glutes, thighs (quadriceps) & hamstrings

Set Up: Begin with body in a stationary lunge position, right leg back, core engaged with hands positioned in front of body or on hips.

Action: In a slow and controlled manner, push off back leg, bringing body into an upward position shifting weight from back leg to front left leg. Hold body in this position for a count and then slowly lower right leg back to starting position. Repeat movement pattern on right leg until set is complete and then switch legs and repeat movement until set is complete.

Single-Legged Bridge

Targeted Muscle: glutes, hamstrings

Set Up: Lie on your back with both feet placed on the ground knees bent, with arms extended by your side.

Action: In a slow and controlled manner, slowly lift right leg off ground, while bridging up on left leg by squeezing your glutes and hamstrings. Hold body in this position for a count and then slowly lower left hip and right leg. Switch legs and repeat movement pattern on the opposite side of your body until set is complete.

***Modified Version:** Keep both feet on ground, and then bridge up.

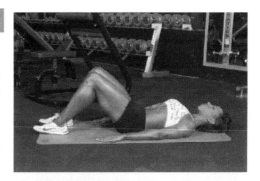

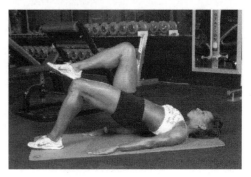

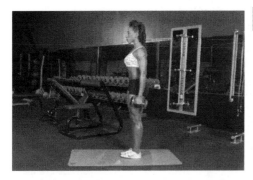

Hamstring Reach

Targeted Muscles: glutes, hamstrings

Set Up: Stand with feet together, slight bend in knees. Arms extended by your side with hands in a neutral position (palms facing inwards towards your body).

Action: While maintaining a slight bend in knees and core engaged, in a slow and controlled manner, bring torso forward reaching dumbbells towards ground and pushing hips back. Hold for a count and then return body back to starting position. Repeat movement until set is complete.

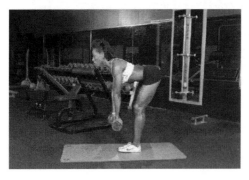

Frog Lifts

Targeted Muscles: glutes, hamstrings

Set Up: Roll forward on stability ball until hips are positioned midway on ball, legs spread apart forming a "V," feet touching ground with arms positioned shoulder width apart.

Action: While keeping legs in "V" position, in a slow and controlled manner, squeeze glutes and move legs in an upward movement towards the ceiling. Hold for a count and then bring legs back to starting position. Repeat movement until set is complete.

*Movement Tip: Keep a slight bend in elbows throughout entire movement. Keep head forward in a neutral position.

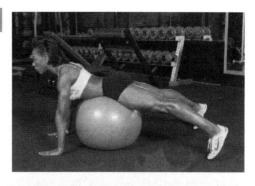

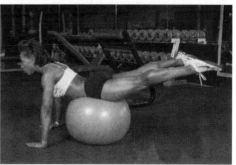

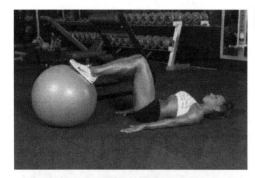

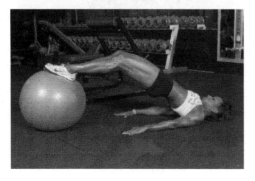

Hamstring Blast

Targeted Muscles: hamstrings, glutes

Set Up: Lay on your back with knees bent, feet flat on stability ball, arms resting near body with palms in a downward position.

Action: In a slow and controlled manner, create an arc movement by pressing feet against ball and lifting hips off ground. Hold for a count and then return body back to starting position. Repeat movement until set is complete.

Curtsy Lunge

Targeted Muscle: quads, glutes, hamstrings

Set Up: Stand with right leg in front and left leg positioned diagonally behind right leg. Slight bend in knees, with hands rested on hips.

Action: In a slow and controlled manner, bend both knees until your thigh is parallel to the ground. Your back knees approaches, but never touches the ground. Hold for a count and then return body back to starting position. Repeat movement until set is complete and then switch front and back legs, repeat movement with opposite stance until set is complete.

*Movement Tip: Make sure knee doesn't go past toes. Keep body in proper alignment with core contracted throughout entire movement.

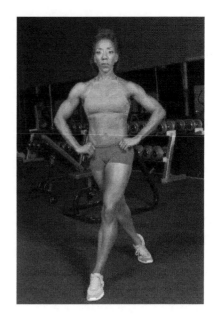

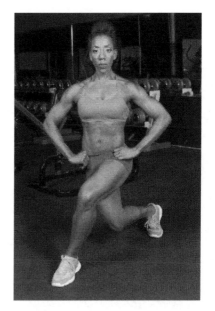

FIT JEWEL

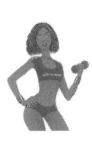

You can't spot reduce to lose weight in a particular part of your legs! You can train smart, consistently and consume healthy well-balanced meals to assist you in losing weight in your legs and your entire body

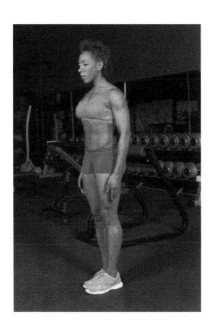

Tick Tocks

Targeted Muscle: glutes, quads (thighs) and hamstrings

Set Up: Stand with feet together, slight bend in knees, arms by your side.

Action: While contracting core, in a slow and controlled manner, bring torso forward reaching both arms in front of body while lifting right leg off the ground. Keep eyes forward and locate a focal point in order to maintain balance. Hold body in this position for a count and then bring body back to starting position. Repeat movement and switch legs. Repeat movement pattern until set is complete.

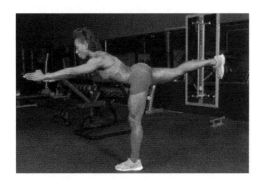

FIT JEWEL

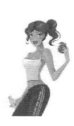

Squat, lunge and bridge for tighter and firmer legs, but don't forget clean eating and regular cardio to help you shed unwanted body fat from your legs. Don't let your hard work go to waste!

Standing Hip Abductions

Targeted Muscles: abductors, glutes

Set Up: Stand with feet together, slight bend in knees. Hands placed on hips or in front of your body.

Action: With slight bend in knee, in a slow and controlled manner, lift leg off ground away from the mid-line or middle of body with knee pointing downward. Keep bend in opposite leg. Hold for a count and then return leg back to starting position. Repeat movement and then switch leg and repeat movement until set is complete with opposite leg.

*Movement Tip: While lifting leg, keep core tight to avoid a shift of weight on supporting leg. If you lack balance or core strength, find an object to hold onto for support.

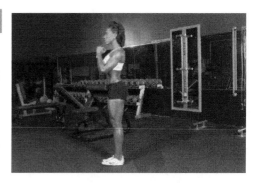

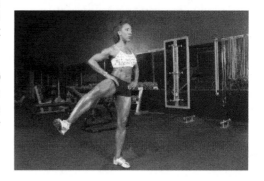

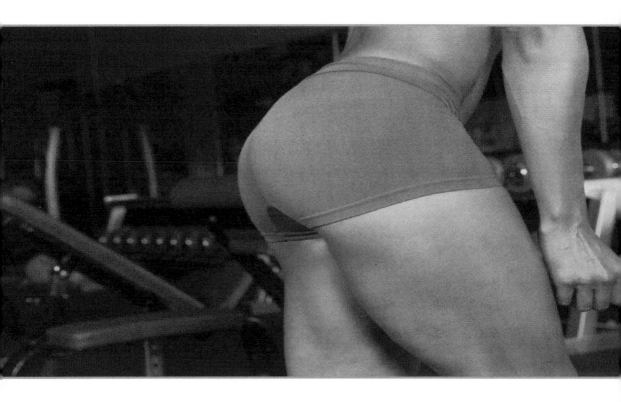

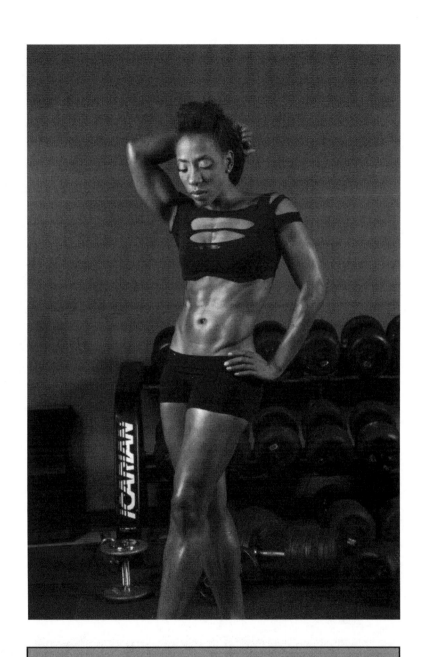

Abdominal Exercises

A Stronger Core, A Stronger You

Your core or abdominal muscles are one of the most important muscle groups in the entire body. Every movement performed requires core stabilization and strength. For some women, this is a challenging area to tone and strengthen. Some women have given birth and as a result have weakened core muscles. On the other hand, some women have jobs that require long hours of sitting and as a result, their core muscles have been weakened and they experience low back pain. Regardless of your profession or whether you are a mother, having a strong core is essential to all of your movements.

Therefore the exercises on the following pages will help you create a more toned and strong core.

Abdominal Exercises

Movement Tip: Keep core contracted while performing each exercise. This will keep body aligned and lessen the chance of injury to your back.

Beginner Level

Exercise	Sets	Repetitions
Knee Taps	2	8-10
Physio-ball reverse knees	2	8-10
Ropes	2	8-10
Walk-Ups	2	8-10

Intermediate Level

Exercise	Sets	Repetitions
Russian Twists with Layout	2-3	12-15
Med-ball Oblique Twists	2-3	12-15
Hanging Abdominal Raises	2-3	12-15
Ropes	2-3	12-15

Advanced Level

Exercise	Sets	Repetitions
Russian Twists with Layout	3-4	15-20
Med-ball Oblique Twists	3-4	15-20
Hanging Abdominal Raises	3-4	15-20
Ropes	3-4	15-20

Targeted Muscles: obliques

Set Up: Begin with feet placed shoulder width apart, slight bend in knees with arms extended overhead while holding medicine ball.

Action: In a slow and controlled manner, contract core and bring right elbow and right knee together, hold for a count. Return to starting position. Repeat movement until set is complete. Switch arm and leg and then repeat movement until set is complete.

*Movement Tip: Keep slight bend in knees throughout entire movement.

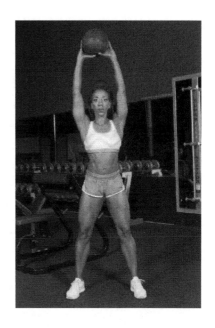

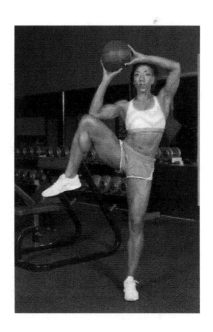

FIT JEWEL

It is essential to remember that although you may strengthen and tone your abdominal muscles with exercise, in order to see your abs, you have to burn the fat surrounding your abs by incorporating healthy well-balanced meals and cardio.

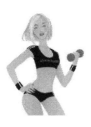

Walk-Ups

Targeted Muscles: abdominals

Set Up: Begin in a push up position, arms shoulder width apart with slight bend in elbows, core tight, lower body in a straight line.

Action: In a slow and controlled manner, step backwards with your hands until your body is in a "V" position. Hold position for a count and then slowly bring body down by moving hands forwards. Repeat movement until set is complete.

*Movement Tip: Only go as far as your natural range of motion will allow.

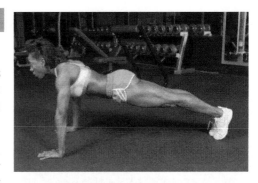

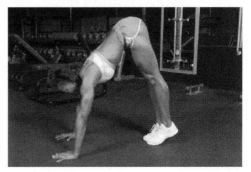

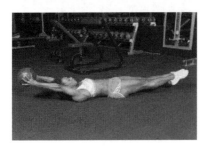

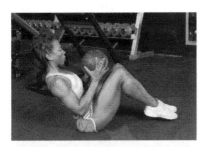

Russian Twists with Layout

Targeted Muscles: abdominals, obliques

Set Up: Place body on mat with feet flat on ground, knees bent, chest up while arms are bent holding medicine ball.

Action: In a slow and controlled manner, bring feet off mat around 2-4 inches. Once stabilized, rotate torso from one side to the other side of the body. After rotation, return torso to starting position, while in this position extend arms overhead and release legs straight in front of your body. Hold for a count and then repeat movement until set is complete.

*Modified Version: Keep feet on ground when rotating and do not perform layout.

Switch-n-Reach

Targeted Muscles: obliques

Set Up: Lie down on a mat with body in a jumping jack position. Arms and legs form an "X".

Action: In a slow and controlled manner, bring right arm towards left leg. Hold for a count and then bring body back to staring position. From starting position, switch arm and leg and repeat movement until set is complete.

Movement Tip: Only lift arm and leg within natural range of motion.

*Modified Version: Keep upper body in same position with legs placed on ground. Instead of bringing arm and leg together, reach opposite arm towards opposite leg by slightly lifting shoulder off mat.

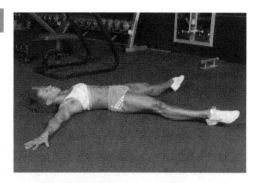

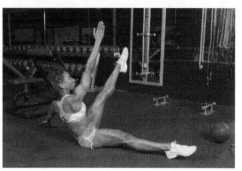

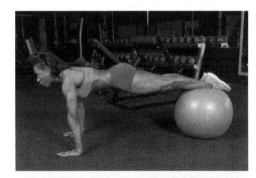

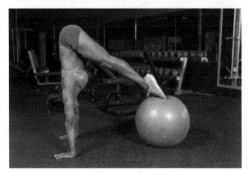

Pike Holds

Targeted Muscles: abdominals

Set Up: In a slow and controlled manner, roll body forward on stability ball until shins rest on ball. Hands are positioned shoulder width apart, core tight and legs in a straight line.

Action: With a slight bend in elbows, in a slow and controlled manner, slowly draw in stomach and lift body into a pike position creating a "V." Hold for a count and then slowly bring body back to starting position. Repeat movement until set is complete.

Windmills

Targeted Muscles: abdominals, obliques

Set Up: While lying on your back, extend both arms out to the side of your body, with left leg fully extended and right knee bent with foot on floor.

Action: In a slow and controlled manner lift upper body off ground in a rotational movement, reaching left arms towards right knee, while right foot lifts off ground. Hold for a count and rotate body back to starting position. Perform movement until set is complete. Switch legs and repeat entire movement on opposite side.

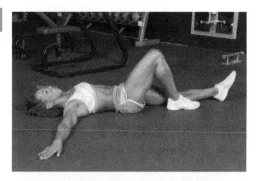

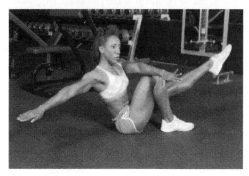

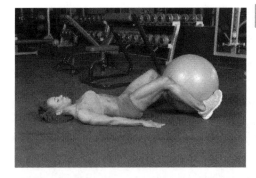

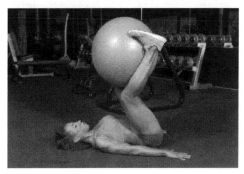

Physio-ball Reverse Knees

Targeted Muscles: abdominals

Set Up: While lying on your back, place physio-ball in between your legs, slightly squeezing your thigh muscles to keep the ball stabilized. Feet are at in a flexed position on ground.

Action: In a slow and controlled manner, engage core and bring feet off ground and knees towards upper body. Hold for a count and slowly bring feet back to ground without allowing feet to fully rest on ground. Repeat movement until set is completed.

Med-ball Oblique Twists

Targeted Muscles: abdominals, obliques

Set up: While lying on your back, with arms extended on ground next to body, knees bent, place medicine ball between thigh muscles, with feet flat on ground.

Action: In a slow and controlled manner, lift feet off ground and rotate hips and knees towards the side of your body. Hold for a count and then bring legs back to the middle of your body and rotate them in the opposite direction and hold for a count. Repeat this movement pattern until set is complete.

Movement tip: Try to keep shoulders on ground when rotating body from side to side. If you can't properly execute movement with medicine ball, remove medicine ball and perform movement without it.

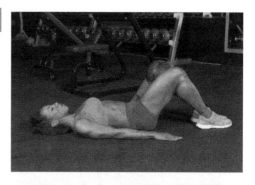

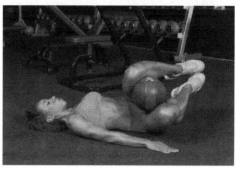

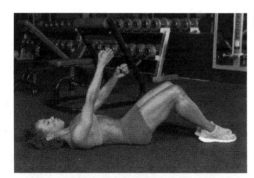

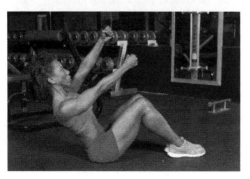

Ropes

Targeted Muscles: abdominals

Set Up: Lay on ground with knees bent, feet flat on floor and arms extended over your head, with one arm staggered over the other.

Action: In a slow and controlled manner engage your core and pretend your hands are climbing up a rope, one hand at a time. Once body is completely off the floor, hold for a count and then slowly reverse your hands climbing back down the rope as your torso returns back to the ground. Repeat movement until set is completed.

Targeted Muscles: abdominals

Set Up: In a slow and controlled manner, jump up or use a bench to grasp and hang from a high bar (Universal Machine) with hands positioned slightly wider than shoulder width apart with and overhand grip, core engaged and body stabilized.

Action: In a slow and controlled manner, slowly raise legs by flexing hips and knees until hips are completely flexed or knees are well above hips. Hold for a count and then slowly return hips and knees to starting position. Repeat movement until set is completed.

Movement tip: When performing this movement do not allow body to swing back and forth. Keep core engaged throughout entire movement and keep slight bend in elbows while hanging from bar.

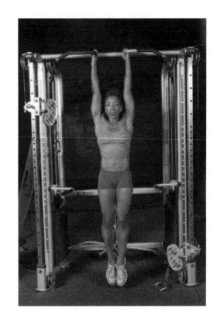

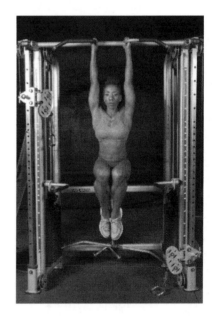

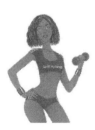

FIT JEWEL

Don't focus solely on getting a 4 or 6 pack. Instead focus on building a strong core that will support your body for the rest of your life!

Curve Sculpting Exercise Tracking Sheet

Use the following sheet to track your exercises, rank intensity levels and mental preparedness for each workout.

Make copies of this sheet and place into a binder to create your own fitness training log.

Date:

Exercise	Sets	Repitions	Rest Time

Mental Fit:

Having a positive attitude about your workout can produce great results. Therefore, before you start your workout, take time to gauge your mental preparation.

Rank your mindset for your workout:
1. I am extremely focused.
2. I am tired, but no more excuses.
3. I will do it because I have to.
4. I am excited about seeing my body change.

Intensity Level:

The amount of effort you put into your workout will determine your overall results.

Rank the amount of effort you put into your workout.
1. I gave 100% - no slacking.
2. I could have pushed harder.
3. I wasn't excited about the workout, but gave it all I had.

From my heart to yours

Chapter

20

Letter from the Heart

What an Amazing Accomplishment!

As you end with this chapter, it is my hope that something you have read has inspired you. I am honored and humbled to have the opportunity to provide you with the tools to help empower your health and your life.

If I told you that I have conquered all of my fears and insecurities, I would be creating a false image of who I am. I have good days and I have days when old thought patterns attempt to invade my mind. It is during these moments that I hold onto the truth of who I am - not based on my appearance, my education or my career. I look at the internal qualities such as my kind spirit, loyalty and other positive qualities that truly define me as a woman.

Maybe all of your life you have been overweight, or maybe you were the one who was always overlooked by those you admired the most. Whatever your story, remember you are important to the world and unique.

Therefore, take each day and continually work on becoming a better version of yourself. It is essential to remember that change does not occur overnight; it's a gradual and sometimes slow, yet rewarding process. In the process of changing, be patient with yourself and allow time for personal growth and physical changes.

Continue to create a support system and don't be afraid to ask for help when you need it. As you grow as a person, you may need to add new people to your support system and that is okay. You're growth is worth seperation from anything and anyone who no longer serves you.

Although I am not with you in person, I carry your struggles and successes in my heart. On the days when you feel alone, remember there are millions of other women who feel the same way you do. Let your light shine so bright that the world will mistaken you for a star.

I look forward to hearing what you have discovered about yourself, and how you are transforming your mind, body and spirit!

Please e-mail me and share your personal story.

Remember, failure is never an option!

Laticia "Action" Jackson

Stay fit, Stay true, Stay you!

Fitness Olympian / 5-Time N.P.C. Fitness Champion

E-mail: Npoweredcoaching@gmail.com

Website: www.npoweredcoaching.com

About the Author
Laticia " Action" Jackson

Laticia "Action" Jackson has over 20 years of experience in the health and fitness field. She holds a Master's Degree in Public Health, B.S. Degree in Exercise Science, A.A. Degree in Human Performance, Certified Personal Trainer, Certified Lifestyle and Weight Management Specialists and Certified Weight Loss Counselor.

She's a 5-Time N.P.C. (National Physique Committee) National Fitness Champion and 2008 Fitness Olympian. She has been featured in over 30 nationally-recognized fitness publications (Oxygen, Muscle and Fitness Hers, Flex, Ironman, Muscular Development) and has made multiple television appearances for stations such as Fox 45/ABC 22 and C.W. 31 as the go-to fitness expert.

As a survivor of domestic violence, it has become her mission to encourage women to love themselves by providing them with the tools to become fit from the inside out. As a Veteran of the U.S.A.F., her discipline and determination has catapulted her fitness and educational career to great heights. She is a member of Delta Sigma Theta Sorority and enjoys volunteering and giving back to her community.

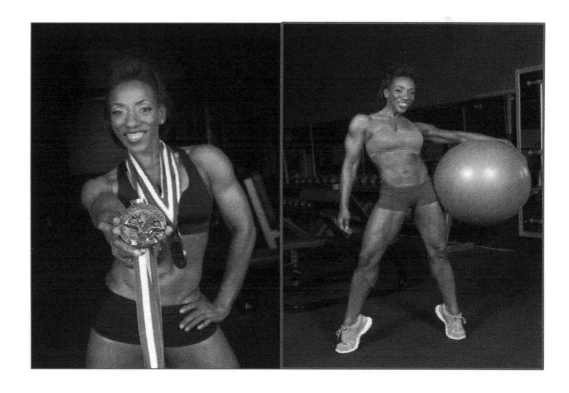

Additional Books Written By Laticia " Action" Jackson

- Goodbye Skinny, Hello Size Healthy- A Woman's Guide to Becoming Healthy, Happy and Satisfied
- Changing the Norm- A Black Woman's Guide To Eating, Feeling and Looking Her Best
- Yes Girls Lift- A Girl's Fitness Guide To Becoming Fit, Confident and Strong
- 10 Days of Inner Discovery- A Path Towards Emotional Healing, Forgiveness and Love
- Don't Complicate It-Basic Nutrition and Healthy Eating Made Simple
- Balanced Nutrition
- Balanced Fitness
- Fit, Tight and Toned- A Black Woman's Roadmap To Sculpting Fit, Tight and Toned Curves
- Fit, Empowered and Unstoppable- A Woman's Fitness Guide To Becoming Her Fittest Most Empowered Self
- Healthy Balanced You- A Woman's Guide To Creating Balance in Her Personal and Professional Life
-

Books Available on Amazon and at
www.npoweredcoaching.com/womenswellnessbooks

Index

Proper Breathing, 126

Protein, 17, 57, 58, 59, 60, 61, 72, 77, 85, 93, 94, 97, 98, 99, 103, 104, 139

Pyramid Pushups, 174, 178

Q

Quadriceps (Front Part Of Leg) Stretch, 152

R

Range Of Motion, 150

Rear Shoulder Raises, 164, 168

Repetition, 135

Resistance Band Extensions, 174, 175

Resistance Bands Curls, 169, 173

Resistance Bands Flyes, 160

Resistance Training, 61, 113, 123, 126, 129, 134, 135, 147, 150, 154, 156, 160, 180

Respiratory, 135

Reverse Lunge With Abductions, 185

Reverse Lunges, 184, 185

Risk Factors, 32

Ropes, 194, 199

Russian Twists With Layout, 194, 196

S

Saturated Fat, 65, 66

Seated Overhead Triceps Extensions, 174, 179

Seated Resistance Band Rows, 161, 162

Set, 114, 128, 135

Shoulder Exercises, 164

Shoulder Rolls, 151

Simple Sugars, 71, 90

Single Legged Bridges, 184

Single-Legged Bicep Curls, 169, 171

Single-Legged Bridge, 188

Single-Legged Chest Press, 156, 158

Snacks, 60, 65, 67, 72, 80, 86, 89, 90

Sodium, 80, 82, 89, 90, 93, 94

Split Stance Hammer Curls, 169, 172

Split Training, 127

Squat Kicks, 184

Squat With Side Kick, 186

Squats, 186

Standing Hip Abductions, 192

Standing Triceps Kickbacks, 174, 177

Straight Arm Extensons, 180

Super Setting, 128

Switch-N-Reach, 197

T

Thoughts, 36, 37, 40

Tick Tocks, 191

Training, 1, 3, 11, 37, 58, 60, 61, 110, 112, 114, 118, 121, 123, 124, 126, 127, 128, 129, 130, 131, 133, 134, 135, 138, 139, 146, 150, 154, 160, 167, 201

Trans Fats, 64, 65

Tricep Exercises, 174

Triceps, 128, 135, 175, 177, 180

Triceps Stretch, 151

Two-Arm Row, 161, 163

Made in the USA
Las Vegas, NV
21 November 2021